ROADS TO RECONCILIATION

ROADS TO RECONCILIATION

Conflict and Dialogue in the Twenty-First Century

———◦◦◦◦◦———

Edited by

Amy Benson Brown and **Karen M. Poremski**

M.E.Sharpe
Armonk, New York
London, England

Library of Congress Cataloging-in-Publication Data

Roads to reconciliation : conflict and dialogue in the twenty-first century / Amy Benson
Brown, Karen M. Poremski, editors.
   p. cm.
 Includes bibliographical references and index.
 ISBN 0-7656-1333-6 (hardcover : alk. paper)
   1. Conflict management. 2. Reconciliation. 3. Violence. I. Brown, Amy Benson, 1966–
II. Poremski, Karen M., 1963–

HM1126.R6 2005
303.6′9—dc22   2004009600

Printed in the United States of America

The paper used in this publication meets the minimum requirements of
American National Standard for Information Sciences
Permanence of Paper for Printed Library Materials,
ANSI Z 39.48-1984.

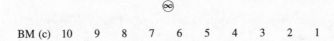

BM (c)   10   9   8   7   6   5   4   3   2   1

Contents

Preface: Our Road to this Volume

The first foreign terrorist attack on American soil happened just as we began to edit this volume of essays on reconciliation. The twin presence of Archbishop Desmond Tutu and former president Jimmy Carter at Emory University in the 1990s led scholars from diverse fields to explore the meaning of reconciliation in their own work. Inspired by Tutu's teaching on reconciliation in South Africa and Carter's experience fostering conflict resolution through the Carter Center, researchers at Emory—along with colleagues at Harvard and the University of Chicago—began to ask questions about barriers to many kinds of reconciliation. We hoped then that gathering their thoughts into this volume would help readers grapple with the multiple and subtle layers of challenges posed by the idea of reconciliation. This seemed to us a project both noble and practical: pursuing reconciliation demands thinking in new ways; it promises the relief of suffering and the freedom born of forgiveness. But on September 11, 2001, the American scale for weighing suffering was recalibrated.

After the attacks, these essays' explorations of the possibilities and limits of reconciliation seemed doomed to be lost in the flood of calls for war and revenge. But within days on our campus, and campuses across the country, there were signs that people were willing to listen as well as react. Non-Muslim students showed support for meetings of the Islamic Student Association. Many professors changed syllabi to help guide students from reaction to analysis. And panel discussions about the tragedy—its causes and consequences—were attended by large and earnest audiences. As we worked with the contributors to prepare this volume, it became clear that the time was growing ripe for serious, cross-disciplinary conversation about the roots of conflict and the complicated process of reconciliation. Reconciliation is an under-researched and under-theorized phenomenon, as Mohammed Abu-Nimer, editor of *Reconciliation, Justice, and Coexistence: Theory and Practice*, has argued. Most of the existing books on reconciliation chronicle attempts to make and sustain peace in countries torn by terrible conflict. As Yaacov Bar-Siman-Tov's recent volume makes clear, however, reconciliation is a multidisciplinary subject that "requires the participation of researchers from a variety of fields." Thus, this collection seeks to chronicle the dynamics of the process of reconciliation as conceived in different scholarly fields, from religion to biology and psychology. Furthermore, we felt that this volume must also speak to issues in light of September 11, if it hoped to inform the contemporary conversation on reconciliation.

An Overview

To define reconciliation, David Whittaker distinguishes it from conflict resolution in his study of steps toward reconciliation in war-ravaged communities. Real reconciliation, he argues, is a process that takes place after conflict resolution and often takes longer than bringing the conflict to an end. Defining genuine reconciliation, though, can be a terribly slippery undertaking. As theologian Steven Kraftchick has noted, the term itself is many-sided, referring to accounts from checkbooks to salvation. He points out that most definitions are either too narrow, describing conditions of one place or problem, or too broad. If reconciliation, for example, is understood simply as any process that unites opposing forces, the term can apply to so many and such diverse situations that coherent analysis of the meaning of reconciliation becomes impossible.

This volume aims to strike a balance between an overly narrow and an impossibly broad understanding of the process of reconciliation. The contexts of the conflicts explored here range from the grand stage of international affairs to the small theater of the individual psyche. Global, religious, and environmental issues recur in many writers' explorations of the roots of international conflicts. Others turn their lenses inward on American culture through analysis of race and class struggles. Unlike other recent books on reconciliation, several writers here also examine psychological turmoil within individuals coping with the aftermath of traumatic conflict—rage, shame, memories of the dead, and the desire for revenge. Despite the diverse types of conflicts these essays explore, they share an understanding that the reconciliation of conflict demands dialogue, self-reflection, and a commitment to the belief in the possibility of significant change. Together, these essays demonstrate that understanding reconciliation requires tearing down the curtain between the personal and the political. They contribute to an appreciation of what Abdullahi An-Na'im describes in his essay as the varieties of "shared vulnerability" experienced by all people. "For some," he writes, "it is the threat of terrorism and other forms of political violence, for others it is political oppression, religious or ethnic persecution, or poverty and disease. The challenge is to see the connections between all these forms of vulnerability, so that we can realize that addressing one form can help alleviate another."

The organization of these essays into sections on religion, science, race and class, and higher education and human rights, described below, does not imply exhaustive coverage of each of those topics. Instead, the sections offer readers a way to map the extensive territory these essays cross. Since the subtleties of language influence the negotiations vital to processes of reconciliation, eminent scholar of rhetoric Wayne Booth opens this volume with a consideration of war rhetoric since September 11 and the history and multiple meanings of reconciliation.

Religion and Reconciliation

The relationship between religion and violent conflict is profoundly ambivalent, as theologian R. Scott Appleby argues in *The Ambivalence of the Sacred: Religion, Violence, and Reconciliation*. While the terrorist attacks of September 11, 2001, will write another chapter in the long history of religion-inspired violence, the religious convictions of believers of diverse faiths—from Mahatma Gandhi to Martin Luther King, Jr. —also have energized movements to build peace.

Because loss and mourning inevitably follow conflict, historian of religion Gary Laderman opens this section by exploring the vexed relationship of the living to their dead. He considers the especially difficult process of grieving and remembrance after September 11 in America. The trauma of loss was compounded for many by the absence of mortal remains of loved ones killed in the terrorist attacks. Drawing on a variety of examples from popular culture, he analyzes the cultural and political significance of the rituals through which Americans remember their dead. Since considerations of religion and reconciliation are linked inextricably to concepts of justice, the next two essays in this section explore alternative understandings of justice.

It has become a commonplace of liberal movements that there can be no peace without justice. It may also be true, however, that there can be no peace with justice, as the director of the Centre for Forgiveness and Reconciliation at Coventry University, Andrew Rigby, has argued. Scholar of religion and violence Theophus Smith explores in his essay why traditional modes of justice often fail to fully resolve conflicts. He argues that in some crimes—especially ones that tend to make the victim feel shame—alternative approaches to justice may bring more satisfaction and peace to the victim and community. In place of familiar codes of justice based on retribution, Smith outlines a system for reconciling offender and victim and restoring both to the larger community. Restorative justice compels offenders to repair the harm they have done, to restore or create ties to law-abiding members of the community, and address some of the causes of their crimes. This alternative vision of justice opens up the possibility of the kind of reconciliation that victim liaison Tammy Krause pursues in death-penalty cases in the United States. Her essay explores the possibilities and limits of reconciliation of victims and perpetrators in her experience in twenty recent legal battles, including her work with *U.S. v. McVeigh*, the trial of American-born terrorist Timothy McVeigh.

Islamicist Richard Martin then moves toward a more global consideration of the roots of violence and possibilities for reconciliation. His essay examines contemporary acts of terrorism associated with militant Islamic extremists as outward manifestations of historically rooted divisions within the Muslim world today. In this final essay of the first section, Martin voices a call repeated by Abdullahi An-Na'im in the volume's closing section: Western cultures must develop a vastly more complex understanding of contemporary Islam.

Science and Reconciliation

Like the essay by Gary Laderman, which opens the religion section, the first essay of this section devoted to scientific perspectives begins with problems rooted in trauma. While Laderman explores the relationship of religious rituals to national identity and culture, psychologist Robyn Fivush examines the dynamics of reconciliation within the traumatized individual. Individual psychological processes can have significant impact on large-scale political outcomes, as David Whittaker has recognized in his study of reconciliation efforts in war-torn countries. Focusing on the psychological impact on college-age students of the September

11th attacks, Fivush explores the similarities of responses to various kinds of trauma and the role of narrative or story-telling in victims' abilities to cope with their experiences. Moving more broadly to the history of human psychology and barriers to reconciliation, anthropologist and psychotherapist Robert Paul then traces the ancient roots of the impulse for revenge.

While the quest for revenge and the psychological drives that thwart reconciliation may lie deep in the history of human development, evolution may also have built into humans certain drives toward resolving conflict peacefully. Eminent primatologist Frans de Waal searches for the origins of human violence in the social interactions of related primates. Through his own research and synthesis of others' work, de Waal shows that among primates the impulse to violent actions coexists with powerful incentives toward cooperation and conflict resolution. Located at the intersection of nature and culture, de Waal's essay provides a fitting segue to the concluding piece of this section by E.O. Wilson, the founder of the field of sociobiology. Wilson links poverty and ecological destruction across the globe to the loss of security from terrorism in the West and calls for a reconciliation of our material needs with responsible environmental practices. He argues that, though we often pit prosperity against environmental preservation, environmental and economic goals are really more intertwined than opposed.

Racial Reconciliation: Theory and Practice in America

This section aims to bring theoreticians of reconciliation together with practitioners in the arena of racial and ethnic justice in American culture. The dynamics of reconciliation have been under-theorized and the relationship between theory and practice neglected, as Mohammed Abu-Nimer has argued. While his volume *Reconciliation, Justice, and Coexistence: Theory and Practice* explores strategies for reconciliation of conflicts around the world, essays in this section focus on the peculiarly American brand of racial conflict.

Using psychoanalytic theory, cultural studies scholar Angelika Bammer unpacks the many meanings of symbols of American patriotism after the September 11th attacks. She suggests the ubiquitous flags and banners declaring "United We Stand" may actually mask the many divisions within a pluralist nation that struggles both to cohere and to accommodate many different forms of "otherness" within it. The history of divisions among blacks and whites in the American South is the focus of an essay by historian Dan Carter. His exploration of the way bias about class complicates our understanding of racial bias leads into anthropologist Johnnetta Cole's analysis of status conflict within racial groups. The former president of Spelman College and current president of Bennett College, Cole explores conflicts within racial groups most often perceived as homogeneous and points to intergroup alliances as ways to break down the black–white paradigm that has dominated discussions of race in the United States. The theoretical and academic approaches to probing race and reconciliation in these essays are complemented in the remaining two pieces by wisdom won from daily political battles. In their essays on their experience of the civil rights movement, both Congressman John Lewis and Reverend Joseph Lowery explore the connections between ethics, social justice, the law, and the potentially transformative powers of theological practice. Important figures in nonviolent political change in America, Lewis and Lowery demonstrate that reconciliation cannot happen in dialogue or theory only, but must happen through action as well.

Higher Education and Human Rights

Since much of the analysis of processes of reconciliation in this volume comes from scholars, the volume concludes with several visions of the role of higher education in promoting the understanding and practice of reconciliation. These essays explore the function of higher education in enabling work toward reconciled communities.

As Whittaker has defined it, a reconciled community is one that "assimilates rather than discriminates, promulgates humane and legal rights, does its best to dissolve alienation and fear, encourages people to share values and develop congenial relationships, and promotes a hope that material benefits will accrue as a product of peaceful transactions and independence." Master teacher Barbara Patterson begins this section by reflecting on the university classroom itself as a kind of community and shares her own practices of reconciliation in the classroom before and after September 11. The essays that follow offer increasingly broad visions of the mission of the university in relation to the larger culture, particularly linking developments at American universities to more global concerns.

Universities are just one source that legal scholar and human rights activist Abdullahi An-Na'im argues should be tapped to support processes that contribute to reconciliation internationally. To move beyond illegal efforts to spur change, like terrorism or vigilante justice, developing countries around the world need structures in place to guarantee both justice and accountability in the resolution of conflicts. Former U.S. president and Nobel Peace Prize winner Jimmy Carter echoes that call for more support for international law and reflects on the role of the university in shaping students to think globally. Broadening and deepening students' understanding of problems that span the world, however, does not require the formulation of any single "grand narrative" of education or reconciliation, as Colgate University president Rebecca Chopp explains. In the concluding essay, Chopp relates the approaches of various contributors to the volume to what she sees as the core mission of the university: the cultivation of intellectual habits of critique, truth-telling, and imagination.

As this book goes to press near the third anniversary of September 11, each day seems to bring news of fresh atrocities from around the world—war, more terrorist attacks, and broken negotiations among those who traveled part of the road toward reconciliation. But as many of the writers in this volume remind us—from their diverse perspectives and in their distinct voices—a different choice is always possible.

Amy Benson Brown
Karen M. Poremski

Bibliography

Bar-Siman-Tov, Yaacov, ed. *From Conflict Resolution to Reconciliation.* Oxford: Oxford University Press, 2004.

Kraftchick, Steven. "Some Reflections on the Difficult Nature and Process of Reconciliation." *Inspiring Reconciliation: Ideas and Practice.* Across Academe no. 2, a series of the Academic Exchange, Emory University, 2001.

Lederach, John Paul. *Building Peace: Sustainable Reconciliation in Divided Societies.* Washington, DC: United States Institute of Peace Press, 1997.

Rigby, Andrew. *Justice and Reconciliation: After the Violence.* Boulder and London: Lynne Rienner, 2001.

Whittaker, David. J. *Conflict and Reconciliation in the Contemporary World.* London and New York: Routledge, 1999.

ROADS TO RECONCILIATION

Introduction

The Rhetoric of War and Reconciliation

Wayne Booth

Preliminary Note, Written September 11, 2002

Everyone who talks about the threat of war faces two conflicting rhetorical temptations: to unite "insiders" for action against the enemy, or to invite "outsiders" into productive discussion. The drive for violent victory now does include a hope for future peace, but the drive for discussion—call it diplomacy, negotiation, genuine listening to the enemy—depends on hope for peace now. Ever since the disaster of September 11, 2001, we have been flooded with the first kind of rhetoric: "This is war and we must win, at any cost." It is war against an "axis of evil," as President Bush put it in his State of the Union address a few months later, employing a phrase that in itself produced a lot of heated controversy between his supporters and those who felt threatened by it.[1] The second kind, the probing for paths to peace, has been far less prominent. While our leaders have exhorted us to join the "war" against the terrorists and—much later—the war against Iraq, one of the three "evil" ones, far too few politicians, let alone journalists or academics, have pled openly for the opposite path: the rhetorical probing for language that might turn enemies into friends—or at least into peaceful dissenters.

This neglect of the rhetoric of reconciliation is not surprising, since we are dealing with terrorists willing to kill themselves in order to kill us. They do not appear to be open to any form of discussion. What hope could President Bush have for a productive dialogue with Osama bin Laden? What would the phrase "the rhetoric of reconciliation" mean to those who piloted the planes to mass destruction? So it was predictable that most of the public declarations would avoid any suggestion of possible reconciliation.

We have thus been presented, by now hundreds or thousands of times, with the assumption that there is only one genuine rhetorical choice: war threats. You, whoever "you" are, must either support "us," the good guys, totally, or suffer total condemnation by "us." If you are not with us, you are "evil." After all, what other choices are there when dealing with suicide bombers?

Such rhetoric risks alienating the vast number of nonterrorists "out there"—those who, for diverse motives, would prefer a quest for peace. Our words (and of course the thinking that leads to those words) have all been designed to unite "us" against "them." Those "out there" who would actually prefer to be our friends but who have multiple allegiances are largely ignored.[2] We seem to be teaching "the world" that there is no point in listening to anybody—except Americans.[3] Yet anyone who really listens to our rhetoric will discover paradox after paradox.

Since this book was planned long before 9/11, much of it addresses conflicts other than international war and peace. In exploring diverse paths to reconciliation in a broad range of subjects, the authors pursue a problem that plagues us not only when war threatens: how to get opponents to listen to one another, in the search for genuine—not hypocritical —reconciliation. In doing so, they perform a key function of rhetoric at its best (too many still think of the word *rhetoric* as referring only to the cheaper forms of persuasion—ranging from sheer verbal trickery to—at best— the prettying-up of arguments derived from less contemptible sources). As I.A. Richards put it in his 1936 celebration of rhetoric, the much neglected *Philosophy of Rhetoric:* "Rhetoric . . . should be a study of misunderstanding and its remedies." [4] Though correcting misunderstanding through genuine listening cannot always produce reconciliation, it is the only alternative to violence or cowardly retreat from the scene.

Just as the word *rhetoric* covers the universal problems of verbal conflict, whether conducted in defensible or indefensible ways, so the term *reconciliation* covers the universal human problem: how to avoid meaningless and destructive conflict of all kinds, verbal and non-verbal. The problems of war language with which I began here are only a fraction of the problem faced in every conceivable kind of conflict: do what you can to conciliate BUT do not sell out in the name of a faked peace and thus enable disastrous error or evil to triumph.

* * *

I can think of no word in our language that covers broader territory than *reconciliation*. Nor can I think of any word that has quite as many synonyms, both in English and in every other language I have consulted. Just consider all the terms we have for our effort to resolve or escape from destructive conflicts. The Internet search engine google.com provides instant evidence for the centrality of the issues faced in this challenging volume. Under:

- "reconciliation"—almost 2 million currently available references;
- "mutual understanding"—almost 2 million references;
- "forgiveness"—almost a million;
- "dispute resolution"—another million;
- "conflict resolution"—another million;
- "agreement reached"—another 2 million.

And so on through "conflict resolved," "conflict managed," "conflict transformation," "conflict settled," "dispute settled," and "arbitration," where I find 1,250,000 references, beginning with "dispute resolution services."

The results of that superficial search through rough synonyms come mainly from what has been written recently. But the fact is that reconciliation has been the center of interest for many from ancient times on, not just in Western culture but surely in all others that have managed to survive. From the Greeks' pursuit of *apokatallasso* through the Romans' pursuit of *reconciliato*, to the twelfth-century French *réconciliation* and the Arabic *Tawfiiq Bayen* (or *Towfeeq Bain*) and on to now, almost all of us—all but the psychopaths—have longed for ways to reduce human conflict. How are we to avoid conflict of the pointless kind that results from misunderstanding on either side? The immense popularity of Homi Bhabha's book, *The Location of Culture*, dramatizes our hunger for paths toward understanding across cultural borders.[5]

Sometimes the word has been used as a synonym for forgiveness of enemies, as Chaucer uses it toward the end of the story of Melibee's shift from revenge to mercy in *The Canterbury Tales* (1387–1400): not really a *rhetorical* reconciliation but a sheer act of charity. Often the word has been used to describe a return to God after sinning, as in Coverdale's "These three nights will we reconcile ourselves with God" (*Tobit*, viii, 4, 1535). In Shakespeare, one usage is to describe reunion of enemies as friends: "Let it be mine honour ... That I have reconciled thy friends and you" (*Titus Andronicus*, I, i, 46, 1594). In *Paradise Regained*, Milton portrays Christ as consigned by Satan to a terrible night, tormented by wind and rain, but remaining "unshaken," as "Fierce rain with lightning mixt, water with fire,/ In ruin reconcil'd" (iv, 413, 1671). In the history of philosophy, the word is often used to describe the attempt to join ideas or deep commitments that seem to clash, as B. Jowett says of Plato: "Without any reconciliation, . . . he speaks at one time of God or the Gods . . . and another time of the good."[6] And so on. "Reconciliation," "reconciled," and their cousins have been key terms for all efforts to draw together whatever has been in danger of falling apart: God and man, friend and foe, rival nations, reason and faith, science and religion, divided political parties, quarreling religions, and on through every conceivable kind of conflict.

That overwhelmingly rich history is hardly surprising. We all know that problems of how to reconcile differences have been with us from the beginning: how to resolve quarrels, how to achieve consensus, how to mend fences, how to restore friendships that have fallen apart, how to interrelate factual claims that seem contradictory, how to re-join, re-conciliate whatever *seems* to clash. Once we were created, whether we believe we came from God or from evolution, we fell into disputes, often into murder or warfare. The Bible dramatizes this point almost from page one. How can Adam and Eve achieve any sort of reconciliation with God? Why can't Cain strive for reconciliation with either Abel or God, instead of killing his brother and being driven out? Why does God throughout the Old Testament so often reject reconciliation with the sinful folks he has created, choosing instead to kill them off? Why does He send the flood rather than organizing a worldwide conference in Babylon? Why does He postpone so long the commandment to seek reconciliation not just with our neighbors but also with our enemies?[7]

The affirmative side of that history is what is reflected in my brief tracing of the word *reconciliation* and its synonyms. None of us would be here if reconciliation had not often triumphed over blind enmity. Though this book cannot possibly cover all of the domains in which reconciliation has worked, or can hope to work, I am not aware of any other book that has offered this breadth of inquiry into so many kinds of conflict.

When we turn to the academy, we see how strongly its history reflects the near universality of both conflict and efforts to resolve conflict productively. Academic "warfare" has been flooded with examples of what might be called anti-reconciliation: the passion for victory no matter what the opponent has to say. It is thus not surprising that we could add to the synonyms for reconciliation I have already listed a host of academic terms for reconciling rival intellectual positions: dialogue, dialectics, hermeneutics, philosophical semantics, philosophical pluralism. Some of these go so far as to land in a dogmatic recommendation to be merely polite to your intellectual enemies, since they are not worth arguing with. Others land in forms of total skepticism about all commitments: it is pointless to seek reconciliation between ideas that are pointless anyway; just be passively indifferent to what the enemies have to say about each other.

The essays in this volume, in contrast, genuinely pursue one or another version of what the concept of reconciliation can lead us to. We should search for:

- "common good" underlying our conflicting values; or
- psychological harmony among rival "selves" that are found within most or all individuals; or
- common humanity beneath seeming racial and gender differences; or
- justice that might conciliate the wealthy with the poor; or
- forgiveness and mercy between criminal offenders and their victims; or
- reconciliation with an environment that we are universally abusing; or
- connections between academic study and the needs of the real world.

And so on, through other areas faced in this book.

For those of us in the academy, the most crucial forms of reconciliation obviously involve finding, or trying to find, common ground shared by contrasting disciplines or intellectual structures or systems: what some call "thought modes," and others, following Thomas Kuhn, label "paradigms." Can physics and biology and mathematics finally be harmonized? Can theologians and philosophers of science come to serious agreement about fundamentals? Can Platonists ever agree with Aristotelians and Spinozists and Kantians and Deweyites? Scientists have from the beginning battled with one another: Is the world made of fire, or air, or water, or atoms, or quanta, or "strings"? Over millennia a few of them have claimed to find a way to harmonize all the views. But most have defended this or that "superior" vision, resisting genuine reconciliation. Kuhn became famous for claiming, as some of his enemies put it, that major scientific positions are essentially *not* reconcilable. Each "paradigm" just dies off as a superior one takes over.[8] Sometimes the dogmatic resistance to reconciliation is defensible: should Einstein simply have bargained with Newton, seeking some middle ground between their views? But often, as in current debates about string theory or the "dreams" of a final scientific "theory of everything," the contenders reveal an overconfident, dogmatic commitment to their own preordained conclusions without really listening to their "enemies."

On the other hand, I believe that these days more scientific and religious thinkers are pursuing reconciliation than ever before. We have a flood of popular books like Edward O. Wilson's *Consilience* and Stephen J. Gould's *Rocks of Ages: Science and Religion in the Fullness of Life* and Ian G. Barbour's *Religion and Science: Historical and Contemporary Issues*. We have hundreds of lesser-known books attempting to reunite "disciplines" that modern research has too often tended to isolate from one another.[9]

To me the most important of these efforts have been those of a few "pluralist" philosophers throughout the last two centuries. How, for example, can we deal with the conflict between a thinker like David Hume, who believes we should *analyze* the world, probing "downward" to discover its hard, irreducible facts and then reasoning "upward" to general truths about them, and a thinker like Plato, who believes that we should start with universal truths, at the top, and reason "downward" to explain the details? And how might we reconcile either of those "greats" with Immanuel Kant's claim that we should start with our *thoughts* about the world? And so on.

The great—and much neglected—philosopher Richard McKeon spent his entire life pursuing a form of systematic pluralism that reconciles the "greats" like Plato and Aristotle and Kant and Hume and Dewey.[10] While such efforts continue, we are flooded with anti-conciliatory works by dogmatists who simply dismiss the "dummies" on the "other side" or by utter skeptics who chant, "It's all pointless."

Wherever we stand on these complex issues—political, philosophical, religious, whatever—it should be clear that the subject of this volume is among the most important of all intellectual challenges. And this challenge forever poses the question of whether we can ever hope for fully successful rhetorical *methods* for achieving reconciliation. If our goal is to avoid or reduce meaningless controversy, or even to achieve full human harmony, how are we to proceed?

For obvious reasons, I cannot answer that question in this Introduction. Nor should any of the authors here be expected to come up with finally decisive positions. But all of them at least implicitly reveal an interest in the one crucial step that underlies all efforts at reconciliation: a serious grappling with the *rhetoric* relied on by disputants. In my view, what we most need—and have needed from the beginning of human conflict to this very day—is a deeper study of the tactics employed by rivals: what I would call—as you may have guessed by now—the diverse "rhetorics of reconciliation."

To suggest that phrase is in itself dangerous. As I have scanned down through about one-tenth of the 10,000 allusions to the phrase "rhetoric and reconciliation" (again on google.com), I am not surprised, only annoyed, to find that a great majority of them are saying, in effect, "We must drop rhetoric, which is merely using trickery in order to win, and embrace rhetoric's opposite, reconciliation." A highly successful book by Samuel George Hines has the title *Beyond Rhetoric: Reconciliation as a Way of Life*.[11] In short, drop the rhetoric and work at reconciliation. Some talk as if they would rule out rhetoric entirely. As one reviewer of a book recently put it, "Anderson slams empty rhetoric and hits back with facts." In other words, get rid of cheap desires to win at all costs—labeled rhetoric—and get down to serious thinking, *anti*-rhetoric.

What those who downgrade "rhetoric" always seem to hope for is some form of discourse that in my definition of the term is still rhetorical: it is an attempt to accomplish some goal through joint communication. At its best, serious rhetoric pursues understanding of the kind that results only when there is genuine *listening* to the opponent's position. Our goal as rhetoricians is to pursue a dialogue that, in contrast to our current militaristic rhetoric, leads the opponent to burst out with something like "Oh, now I understand your position." Or at least, "Oh, *now* I can see that we can get somewhere as we talk together."

As a lifetime student of rhetoric in that broader sense, I have always been annoyed by the pejorative reductions, but I know that they are not going to go away. "Mere" rhetoric in the nasty sense will always be employed by those who hope to avoid reconciliation, or even hope to destroy the enemy. Various unfair kinds of "mere" rhetoric are being employed harmfully throughout the world. At this moment—whenever it is that you are reading this sentence—violence threatens many corners of the world. The rhetoric is shouted, often in total sincerity, by contestants who are sure that they have the whole truth, that the opponents are benighted, or even evil. If rhetoric means only "manipulation of language to win," it will always be the enemy of reconciliation.

But if we pursue "the rhetoric of reconciliation" as something like, "how the deep listening to and examination of one another's rhetorical moves can correct misunderstanding and yield reconciliation," then what we need—will this sound dogmatic?—is continued revival of deeper and deeper forms of that rhetoric of reconciliation. By teaching ourselves and our opponents how to *listen* to our rival rhetorics, we can win the one genuine victory: reconciliation.

For now, I can only suggest that readers ask the following four questions as they read each of these challenging essays. Some of the authors may feel offended by the intrusion of one or another of these questions, but as I pursue what I have sometimes labeled "rhetorical harmony," or even the ugly term "rhetorology," I am convinced that every author or reader in all subjects finally needs to probe all four questions.

I. What is this author's *definition* of the "combatants" who are quarreling, or openly seeking reconciliation, or should be seeking it, and what is the *definition* of the "subject" being quarreled about? Is there an underlying basic view of human nature and the matter debated here, a definition that presupposes success or failure in reconciliation efforts? Is the assumption, for example, that we humans are basically, inherently, committed to conflict, and that our goal is always just to win? Or are we creatures who at the deepest level hope for some kind of truce or diplomacy about this subject?

II. What are the author's central *principles or presuppositions* about the "nature of things" or "the world" or "the whole of nature" or "God's universe"—the scene in which conflict occurs? What assumptions about "the whole of reality" underlie the inquiry?

III. Which of the author's notions of the *methods of discussion* are most likely to yield reconciliation? The history of thought exhibits immense controversy among philosophers about just which methods are philosophically defensible. What does this author see as the appropriate or decisive sources of proof, and where does he or she see the opponent or opponents as standing?

IV. What is the author's primary goal, end, purpose? How would he or she answer the question "So what?" Fortunately, this last one when asked throughout this book will yield an answer shared in more or less the same way by all of the authors: the *goal* of the inquiry *is* reconciliation and finding ways to achieve it. A primary curse of our lives is our impulse to follow Cain and strike blows at targets without first trying to understand them. We too often shoot at targets that are not really there, and thus we destroy "enemies" who might otherwise have become friends. In contrast, all the authors here are at least in this one respect practicing the rhetoric of reconciliation.

I do not have to tell you that even the most rigorous attention to these four questions, which I borrow from McKeon, who borrowed them from Aristotle—questions of definitions, principles, methods, and purposes—has its limitations, just as even the most devout pursuant of reconciliation can only *sometimes* achieve it. No one can ask the four questions when dealing with terrorists who do not even issue a statement about why they made the attack. When an angry father and son charge onto the baseball field and start pounding a coach, and the coach's team rushes out and starts pounding the two attackers (as happened on September 19, 2002, in Comiskey Park in Chicago), reconciliation is killed by sheer blind hatred, on both sides. If neither side will listen, nor choose to speak as if hoping the other side *will* listen, we can hope for nothing more than violence, or even warfare.

We have no way of knowing whether the promise of the most optimistic religious reconciliators will ever be achieved: peace on earth and good will toward all people, reconciliated by or with God. It is sadly true that many among those now referred to as enemies will never have learned the rhetoric of reconciliation, and will never really listen to us even if we drop the war rhetoric and pursue other paths. It is also sadly true that too many of "us" feel self-righteous when we refuse to listen the "evil" ones. Perhaps all we can hope for is a widespread reduction in the pointless aiming at targets that do not even exist.

Yet when we consider how many stupid, cruel conflicts of America's past have been mainly resolved in the twentieth century—just how much conciliation has occurred among us "WASPS" and Jews and African Americans, Latinos and Asian Americans—perhaps we should feel some

optimism. Not just individuals but whole cultures can learn how to practice the rhetoric of reconciliation—if they are willing to work at it.

Dare I hope that by the time this Introduction is in print, America
will have avoided World War III, while still managing to cope with
terrorism?

Notes

1. Many thought he had referred only to three nations, North Korea, Iran, and
Iraq. But his axis was much broader: "States like these [three], *and their terrorist
allies*, constitute an axis of evil, arming to threaten the peace of the world" (my
italics).

2. As I revise here on September 11, 2002, I have felt almost depressed by how
the media concentration on the anniversary—in one sense entirely appropriate—has
almost totally neglected the problem of working to understand the perspective of the
"outsiders," not just the would-be terrorists but all those potential friends—and
enemies—all over the world. We have spent our time arousing our defensive passions, while ignoring others' reasons—valid and invalid—for mistrusting our policies. Only a rare item here and there reveals an author who has really worked at the
problem of *listening*.

3. Yet as I revise a bit later, I see some reasons for encouragement, as Senators
Kennedy and Durbin and Daschle and Byrd and a few others are speaking out.

4. *The Philosophy of Rhetoric*, ed. John Constable (London: Routledge, 2001),
p. 1. (Orig. 1936).

5. Despite the density of Bhabha's language, every careful reader finds that he
is wrestling with the problems of *cultural* reconciliation. For example: "It is in the
emergence of the interstices—the overlap and displacement of domains of difference
—that the intersubjective and collective experiences of nationness, community interest, or cultural value are negotiated. How are subjects formed 'in-between,' or in
excess of, the sum of the 'parts' of difference (usually intoned as race/class/gender,
etc.)? How do strategies of representation or empowerment come to be formulated
in the competing claims of communities where, despite shared histories of deprivation and discrimination, the exchange of values, meanings and priorities may not
always be collaborative and dialogical, but may be profoundly antagonistic, conflictual
and even incommensurable?" (New York: Routledge, 1994), p. 2.

6. *The Dialogues of Plato*, 2d ed., IV, 2 (New York: Scribner's Sons, 1871).

7. I must resist the temptation to trace the history of efforts to prove that when
the Bible commands us to love our "neighbors," it intends the word to cover every
human being. For a fine brief tracing of "love thy neighbor" in the Hebrew Bible,
see Paul Mendes-Flohr, "A Postmodern Humanism from the Sources of Judaism,"
Criterion: A Publication of the University of Chicago Divinity School, Vol. 41 (Spring
2002): 18–23.

8. Thomas Kuhn, *The Structure of Scientific Revolutions* (Chicago: University
of Chicago Press, 1970. Orig. 1962). The first edition was misinterpreted by some
as a claim against any form of solid scientific truth; Kuhn worked hard to clear up
that problem in his "Postscript" to the second edition.

9. A striking example is Alan G. Gross's *The Rhetoric of Science*, in which he argues that every scientific step, regardless of how empirical, is dependent on rhetorical proofs; rhetoric and science are, for him, ultimately reconcilable. But, as one might predict, Gross's splendid book has produced probably more controversy than genuine reconciliation (Cambridge, MA: Harvard University Press, 1990. 2d ed., 1996).

10. See *Selected Writings of Richard McKeon*, vol. 1: *Philosophy, Science, and Culture*, ed. Zahava McKeon and William Swenson, especially the essay "The Uses of Rhetoric in a Technological Age: Architectonic Productive Arts" (Chicago: University of Chicago Press, 1999). Or have a look at a masterful effort at philosophical reconciliation, Walter Watson's *The Architectonics of Meaning: Foundations of the New Pluralism*, 2d ed. (Chicago: University of Chicago Press, 1993).

11. Valley Forge, PA: Judson Press, 2000.

Part I

Religion and Reconciliation

Rites and Remembrance

Living with the Dead of September 11

Gary Laderman

How to live with the dead? All human societies draw on a variety of symbolic and ritual resources to answer this question. Death, like birth, is one of the most natural, biologically inevitable events in human life. But the experience of losing a loved one disturbs the most fundamental ties that bind person to person in any community. These relations are reaffirmed during funeral rituals soon after death for sure, but they are also maintained long after the dead have been put in their final resting place through public ceremonies that celebrate their memory and private acts of remembrance that keep them present. The spirits of the dead and their physical bodies thus offer profoundly significant but sadly incompatible images of life after death. Often those spirits seem to return to haunt the living, console the bereaved, or bring timeless knowledge back to inhabitants of this world, while the physical bodies may be briefly displayed for some form of public viewing, then quickly ushered out of sight before ultimate disintegration. The work of culture is to reconcile these two images, make sense of the gap between them, and find ways to live with the difference.

But some deaths disturb the living more than others. The deaths of popular political and cultural figures, of infants and children, of individuals who die tragically and without purpose, of suicides who choose to prematurely end their lives, and of victims of war or terrorism—in these kinds of circumstances, efforts by the living to meaningfully reconcile themselves to the loss of life prove much more difficult and require more innovative and imaginative strategies than those readily available in the cultural reserve. From the unprecedented televised funeral of John F. Kennedy in 1963 and the chilling televised murder of Lee Harvey Oswald by Jack Ruby the same weekend as the funeral, to the recent *Columbia* shuttle disaster, television and popular culture in general have mediated the encounters between the living and the dead. This is especially true in the most horrific and ritually challenging of circumstances: those in which there are irretrievable bodies.

Contemporary American popular culture is particularly suited to serve as the medium for these encounters. It has always integrated the facts of death into the fabric of everyday life. Contrary to the common accusations leveled against popular culture—that it is frivolous entertainment, mindless distraction, or superficial idol-worship—this dimension of public life is the primary arena in which Americans negotiate the meanings and values that rule their lives. Church services, political rallies, parades and processions, and other familiar public settings once assumed the gravely serious responsibility of enacting rituals and enunciating meanings that made sense of troubling deaths to grieving Americans. But now film, music, television, news media, cyberspace, magazines, advertising, and other cultural pathways through popular American preoccupations determine how tragic times are processed and understood.

This essay explores some of the cultural work of making sense of death in the aftermath of the 9/11 attacks, focusing primarily, though not exclusively, on the devastation in New York City. In the immediate aftermath of the attacks came the urgent, deeply sorrowful task of responding to mass death without access to the bodies of those lost in the Twin Towers. Americans witnessed a variety of special media reports, concerts, and public memorial services that salved some of the collective sadness. Almost a year after this loss, the popular release of *The Rising*, an album inspired by the events of that day by one of America's best known and most beloved rock stars, Bruce Springsteen, offered a vision of reconciliation with death and the dead that resonated with the grieving public. Finally, this essay looks back on the media coverage of the events surrounding the first-year anniversary of the attacks, briefly analyzing how the news media framed the collective and cultural memory of the attacks.

Horror and Fascination: The Days and Weeks Following September 11

On September 11, 2001, terrorists made their fateful and fatal attack on the United States, using commercial airplanes as bombs to destroy New

York City's Twin Towers and part of the Pentagon in Washington, D.C. If one of the planes had not crashed in Pennsylvania, the White House or the Capitol might also have been hit. The days and weeks after these events were surreal at times, filled with anguish, disbelief, astonishment, sadness, outrage, and anxiety. The terrorist act against the nation was an awesome spectacle of death and destruction, an extraordinary morning of horror that annihilated thousands of bodies in vital national centers by lunchtime. The successful nature of the attack, the chilling impact it had on the life of the nation in the months after, and the declaration of war on terrorism by President George W. Bush will no doubt change the course of American history.

The loss of these innocents, the incineration of their bodies and their irretrievable condition in the ruins, will leave scars in American life that both transcend history and propel it forward. The dead will remain eternally present in our memories and be seen as models of virtue and heroism —they are the first martyrs of the twenty-first century—just as their blood and ash, mixed with concrete and steel, will become valuable relics in the cultural efforts to memorialize the atrocities of 9/11 in a fitting way.

As many commentators have repeatedly asserted, what took place on that day was unprecedented in American history. The only remotely comparable events are the terrorist attack in Oklahoma City, which led to the execution of Timothy McVeigh, and the surprise attack on Pearl Harbor, which led to America's full involvement in World War II and the eventual dropping of the atomic bomb on two cities in Japan. Certain individual tragic deaths have made a dramatic impact on the national psyche, including those of Abraham Lincoln, John F. Kennedy, Martin Luther King, Jr., and space shuttle *Challenger* astronaut Christa McAuliffe. After these figures died, Americans found new and innovative ways to memorialize and celebrate them. Public displays of communal mourning, sometimes officially organized, sometimes more spontaneous expressions of shared loss, often brought large groups of people together across class, gender, religious, and racial lines. In all cases, these can be considered public rites of civil religion, an expression of the national spirit that periodically transforms the nation into a church with common rituals, shared myths, and vital symbols. Americans were united in grief, and by that very unity, communities then were able to transcend the sad, terrible circumstances of these individual deaths.

The cold, brutal facts of September 11th's acts of terror, and the vast bloodbath in their wake, will not be easy to overcome for those most directly affected, nor for the rest of us, psychically marked by the images, news accounts, and nightmares of hijacked planes and exploding buildings. For many, institutional religion provides the most gratifying answers to the horrible questions associated with larger metaphysical issues related to evil and suffering, punishment and forgiveness. But when it comes down to the physical, most religious traditions take the body seriously at death and require its presence—seen or hidden, close or distant—to address essential questions about the ultimate meaning of life, unavoidable truths about identity, and the crucial value of social relations among the living and between the living and the dead.

Media coverage of 9/11 immediately began to focus on this dilemma for a number of different religious communities, often emphasizing the profound importance of having a body in the ritual ceremonies to say a proper farewell. Within three weeks, the *New York Times* ran the story "Rites of Grief, Without a Body to Cry Over." The article explains that hundreds of families had been "robbed . . . of intimacy" and "cheated out of . . . rituals" because of missing bodies. "Having the deceased dressed in her favorite clothes for a Catholic wake, scattering ashes in a river for a Hindu ceremony, reading prayers at the Jewish cemetery, cocooning the body in a white shroud for a Muslim burial . . . none of them are possible." The article goes on to offer heartbreaking examples of families needing to improvise, to rely on photographs or other memorabilia that do not seem enough or quite right for the occasion.[1] A *San Francisco Chronicle* article mentions Muslims, Buddhists, and Jews, all ritually enfeebled without access to whole bodies of the dead. It also covers former mayor Giuliani's desperate and disturbing gesture to provide survivors with something material from the Twin Towers: an urn with ash and other materials from the site of destruction.[2]

In the face of such an unparalleled attack, and in the midst of such incomparable ritual confusion, desperate signs of meaning-making and communal action began to emerge from the ground up, so to speak. Without the usual cultural scripts to work from, people close to the disaster site did what most communities do in trying times: improvise. A *New York Times* report at the end of September noted a "sad and inevitable change" that took place at Ground Zero. More and more family members who lost a loved one began to visit the site—so many that a separate ferry between midtown and the financial center had to be set up—and leave mementos, flowers, personal notes, photographs, and other intimate objects that connected them with their dead. "Hundreds of people . . . have quietly toured what they now reluctantly regard as a final resting place—perhaps the only semblance of a graveyard the 5,000 or so lost will ever know."[3] For many affected by this nightmare, a pilgrimage to the site brought them physically closer to their missing relations, now and forever intermingled with rubble and ash.

Without identifiable bodies to ground our responses, and lacking familiar funeral rituals that can provide an orderly manner in which to dispose of the dead individually, close family members and all Americans were left with literally nothing to focus their hearts and minds on. Instead, the wrenching sight of homemade flyers with pictures of the missing and the common memorial street scenes displaying personal expressions of grief began to appear. The photographs, so many pictures of life, of individuals once in the midst of life, provided visual evidence for specific identities lost in the debris and spoke to the deep yearning to have something more than an image to commemorate the death. In ordinary circumstances, the dead body cries out for ritual, and whether it is ultimately cremated and dispersed to the wind, embalmed and put on display, or cared for by community members and placed in the ground, Americans rely on its temporary presence to properly and meaningfully say good-bye.

Some media outlets covered the reaction of local funeral directors in the days after the horrible events, the very people normally charged with managing the body's temporary presence after death and before it vanishes. On September 22, *Newsweek* carried the story "Final Respects: New York's Funeral Industry Prepares for an Onslaught." In it, the reader learns about companies shifting casket inventories closer to New York City, state agencies surveying open cemetery space in the surrounding areas, and medical authorities providing sobering details about the small number of bodies recovered and the disturbingly large number of unidentifiable body parts. The piece explains that even though bodies were missing, Americans who lost close relations were turning to America's funeral directors to assist in planning the appropriate ceremony. It also mentions that recent historical changes in the funeral industry should prepare them for the wide variety of celebrations and ceremonies desired by devastated family and friends: "Still, it helps that in recent years, funeral etiquette has loosened up, and funeral directors are more accustomed to hosting nontraditional memorial services. 'We used to think of funerals as just tending to the dead,' says Vincent O'Conner of the Dennis O'Conner Funeral Home in Rockaway, N.Y. 'Now we see them as an opportunity to celebrate the person's life.'"[4]

This effort to "celebrate the person's life" and find appropriate ritual actions and words to transform the carnage at Ground Zero into dignified moments honoring the dead did not end in funeral homes. Another significant form of cultural improvisation that sought to appropriately and honorably respond to this instance of mass death appeared in the pages of the *New York Times*. "Portraits of Grief" began as a journalistic effort to assist in the large-scale efforts to identify the missing; often working from the homemade flyers that blanketed the city in the days following the attack, journalists for the *Times* printed sketches, or short biographies, of the missing. It soon evolved into something more than a supplemental obituary page and assumed a prominent place in the *Times*, eventually earning the paper one of its six Pulitzer Prizes for coverage of the terrorist attack. Identifying a distinction between the portraits of the dead from 9/11 and regular obituaries, *Times* metro editor Jonathan Landman stated: "Portrait is a good word—snapshot's a good word. Obituary is a bad word." A *Times* journalist elaborated about the content: "Not what schools they went to, how many children they had, what job promotions they'd had. But more their passions, the things they loved, funny stories about them."[5]

In the weeks and months following 9/11, "Portraits of Grief" emerged as a profoundly moving, culturally compelling social artifact that did not simply offer readers dramatic, often poignant biographies of individuals who died in the Twin Towers. It also served a religious function that extended beyond the circle of relations most affected by the day's events, resonating with traumatized Americans throughout the nation and generating critical social solidarity inspired by the fate of the dead. One reporter writing about the cultural impact of the portraits referred to them as a "national shrine": "Reading 'Portraits of Grief' became a ritual for people nationwide. In hundreds of e-mail messages and letters to the *Times*, readers said they read them religiously, rarely missing a day. For some, it was a way of paying homage. Others said it was a means of connecting, a source of consolation. . . . One reader, a lawyer in Manhattan, called reading the profiles 'my act of Kaddish.'"[6] In the aftermath of an extraordinary day of death and destruction, this unexpected, but ultimately apposite, innovation in public mourning ritually brought the absent dead into living society; though without bodies, the faces, personal stories, and reminiscences helped to partially overcome the circumstances of their deaths and give life to their spirits.

City in Ruins: Living with Phantoms

In July 2002, Bruce Springsteen released his first album with the E Street Band in over fifteen years. *The Rising* was a huge commercial and critical success, ultimately selling millions of albums and garnering three Grammy Awards. Its success was due in part to the legion of fans who had waited over five years for a new studio album from Springsteen and to the popular appeal of its robust but wide-ranging musical styles. More than anything, though, its popularity is based on the sorrowful presence of the dead from 9/11 in most of the songs on the album, phantoms simultaneously inspiring one of America's most celebrated musical performers and haunting the lives of Americans who still have not adequately put them to rest. While some of the songs were written before 9/11, the album in its entirety brings together elements of rock, gospel, soul, and funeral dirges to produce a work that is both mournful and celebratory in its engagement with the horror and death of that day.

Music proved to be a popular medium for consoling Americans reeling from the September attacks. Musical tributes and public concerts to benefit bereaved families appeared on the cultural scene right away, including "America: A Tribute to Heroes," a telethon devoted to raising money for the September 11th Fund. It featured Springsteen as the opening performer, singing "My City in Ruins," the closing track of *The Rising*, and a song he had written before 9/11 about the economically troubled times of his old haunting grounds, Asbury Park, New Jersey.

The song, however, was eerily appropriate for the post-9/11 psychological landscape of New Yorkers—and all Americans—traumatized in the aftermath of terrorist strikes. With lyrics like, "There's a blood-red circle on the cold, dark ground/And the rain is falling down, the church door's thrown open, I can hear the organ's song/But the congregation's gone" and a chorus that inspires the listener to "rise up, come on rise up," the song clearly struck a chord with the American public, who struggled to come to grips with nightmarish images of the towers crashing to the ground. Springsteen's music, along with that of other musical performers, provided Americans with an alternative cultural language to the political rhetoric emanating from public figures to help process and reflect on the day's events.

Indeed, Springsteen himself immediately turned to music after watching the events unfold before his eyes on television. The first two songs he wrote in the weeks following 9/11 were "Into the Fire" and "You're Missing," two of the more evocative songs on the album. The former, written from the perspective of a firefighter climbing the stairs in one of the towers, begins: "The sky was falling and streaked with blood/I heard you calling me, then you disappeared into the dust, up the stairs, into the fire." Moving from the sadness of the doomed hero, who "walked into the smoky grave," to the spiritual uplift of the chorus, "May your strength give us strength/May your faith give us faith/ May your hope give us hope/May your love bring us love," Springsteen conveys both the tragic and the transcendent, the suffering and the hope, that offers listeners a frame of reference to construct a meaningful and humane response to the chaos indelibly marked in American historical memory.

While "Into the Fire" encompasses both blues, in the verses, and gospel in the chorus, "You're Missing" wallows in the mournful, heartbreaking reality of loss and despair for families who must live with the glaring absence of loved ones. "Picture's on the nightstand, TV's on in the den/ Your house is waiting, your house is waiting, for you to walk in, for you to walk in/But you're missing, you're missing." This is a disturbing, uncompromising lament for the dead, an attempt to empathically enter the domestic world of grieving survivors who will be reminded of their lost relations for the rest of their lives. The song, in this case, does not provide spiritual uplift or hopeful transcendence. It ends on a dramatically depressing, spiritually ambiguous note: "God's drifting in heaven, devil's in the mailbox/Got dust on my shoes, nothing but teardrops."

Like the rest of the nation, Springsteen spent a good deal of time reading the *New York Times* obituaries that eventually became "Portraits of Grief." He noticed that a number of these portraits made reference to him; his songs were played at memorial services for the dead, and biographies of individuals who perished in the attacks often noted that Springsteen, who had not known these individuals, was a deeply meaningful presence in their lives. In a strange way, Springsteen was a phantom presence for them before they died, a figure who had no personal relationship with them but who yet occupied a special place in their lives and who animated a significant element of their identities.

After 9/11, Springsteen found inspiration in these dead, phantoms now animating a significant element of his musical identity. Indeed,

Springsteen eventually contacted family members of some victims who had included him in their portraits, in order "to flesh out the intimacies of Sept. 11," in the words of a *TIME* cover story on Springsteen in August 2002. He literally got to know the dead before writing the bulk of the album, and quickly produced and then released it to the public—a timetable dramatically opposed to his usual work ethic. This complicated familiarity with the victims, knowing something of their personal histories, quite a bit about the horrible circumstances in which they died, and barely anything about the suffering endured by the living, is expressed through the range of musical styles on the album and the diverse emotional responses conveyed by the lyrics. They range from the biblically informed cry for vengeance in "Empty Sky"—"On the plains of Jordan/I cut my bow from the wood/Of this tree of evil/Of this tree of good/I want a kiss from your lips/I want an eye for an eye/I woke up this morning to the empty sky"; to the more stoic resignation that comes with day-to-day living in "Lonesome Day"—"House is on fire, viper's in the grass/A little revenge and this too shall pass/This too shall pass"; to the burning religious dedication expressed in the bonds between the dead and the living in "The Rising"—"There's spirits above and behind me/Faces gone black, eyes burnin' bright/May their precious blood bind me/Lord, as I stand before your fiery light."

Springsteen writes about the power of the dead and their elemental role in social relations among the living, a role thrown into dramatic relief after 9/11. As an early review of *The Rising* in *Entertainment Weekly* concluded, "'The Rising' is a ghost story, but it's more, too—past and present, celebration and wake—and few others could have pulled it off."[7] The album is an artistic accomplishment for sure, but it also taps into deep-rooted, cross-cultural concerns about the boundaries between the living and the dead, and, at least in one song, "Worlds Apart," hints at the potential dangers if the boundaries are crossed: "May the living let us in, before the dead tear us apart." Whether they appear as spirits, in memories, or as just missing, Springsteen is desperately trying to account for the 9/11 dead, to reconcile himself to the phantoms that will likely haunt him and his listeners for the rest of their lives.

In interviews, Springsteen has also acknowledged a crucial, if not *the* crucial, social fact about the unspeakable horror of the day already mentioned: annihilated bodies, leaving nothing with which grieving friends and family members can ground their ritual impulses. In the August *TIME* cover story, Springsteen says: "Loss is about what you miss. . . .

You miss a person's physical being—their skin, their hair, the way they smell, they way they make you feel. You miss their body. When my father died, my children wanted to touch him, to touch his body. And the kids got something out of it. The people in this situation, you know, they aren't going to get that."[8]

Springsteen contemplates the profound dilemma faced by family members and friends without material traces of their close relations who perished in the attacks. While this provides the underlying reality that haunts much of the album, the singer searches for momentary points of intimacy, connection, and reconciliation with the dead. Indeed, in one of the more rambunctious and hopeful songs on *The Rising*, Springsteen assumes the persona of Death to establish a relationship with the dead. On "Further On (Up the Road)," Springsteen sings, "Got on my dead-man suit, and my smilin' skull ring/My lucky graveyard boots, and a song to sing." In spite of this level of identification with death, however, there remains the possibility of transcendence, or overcoming human finitude under any circumstances for Springsteen: "one sunny morning, we'll rise I know."

National Regeneration One Year Later

Historian Sidney Mead once published a book about America called *The Nation with the Soul of a Church* (1975). While he was referring to certain key theological principles animating the political life of the republic, the spiritual life of the nation is clearly tied to another fundamental truth about the rise and spread of Christianity: many churches were built directly above, and were consecrated by, holy relics associated with the graves of early Christian martyrs—an intimacy between the living and the dead commonly found in religious cultures throughout the world. In American public culture a year after the 9/11 attacks, the deep and profound connections between the dead and the "nation with the soul of a church" were evident in news media accounts of local and national efforts to make sense of this trauma.

Media coverage of the literally thousands of commemorations around the country marking the first anniversary of the terrorist attacks against the United States highlighted a distinctive, and deep-rooted, feature of national religious life: the invocation of the figurative and literal presence of the dead regenerates social solidarity in communal rituals as well as solitary spirituality in private reflections. News reports on September 11 and 12, 2002, noticed the undeniable connections between death, religion, and national life. At first glance, most journalists remained focused on local acts of public worship and memorialization, individual stories of tragedy and triumph, and speculative musings about how, or if, 9/11 changed American life. But upon closer inspection, it becomes clear that all of the individual and collective efforts by Americans to face the vivid and visceral memories of that day zeroed in on the dead and what their deaths mean to the nation.

The *Houston Chronicle*'s approach illustrates the point. On September 12 it covered many of the local events commemorating the anniversary in a story headlined: "Thousands crowd places of worship to find solace." Most of those interviewed expressed the need to give the dead—and their God—their due, an especially difficult task given the brutal circumstances of the day. Like so many articles, the *Chronicle* story wove the lives of individuals struggling with the memories of these vicious acts into the larger tapestry of national community and collective remembering. "Thousands of Houstonians joined Americans nationwide in crowded houses of worship and outdoor ceremonies Wednesday, seeking community and healing. 'It is a day that is unforgettable,' said Paula DeLeon Vargas, who rode a bus to Sacred Heart Co-Cathedral to pray. 'It is for all the people who were lost. For all the families that God give them fortitude. God is the only one who can give them the strength to continue.'"[9]

On September 12, the *Buffalo News* ran the story "A call to remember" by Phil Fairbanks. Here too, the expressions of personal sorrow as well as forms of public ritual in and around Buffalo that bound community members together—and that bound Buffalo to the rest of the nation—radiated from memories of the dead, memories many believed would transform the nation. "Everywhere you went, people spoke of the need to honor those who died and," Fairbanks writes, "even more important, to never, ever forget what happened on Sept. 11, 2001, the day that changed all of us—forever."[10] Journalists exposed the vital links between these dead and national identity, a meaningful and familiar pattern in American history even under these extraordinary circumstances.

CNN also reported on widespread efforts to commemorate the dreadful day by bringing the dead back into national consciousness through ritual acts of memory and private moments of silent reflection. In a roundup headlined "Americans remember 9/11 in many different ways" from September 11, 2002, the story was ritual diversity. Descriptions of a wide variety of ritual activities around the country, such as a moment of silence at 9:11 P.M. by Major League Baseball, a riderless horse parading in Helena, Montana, or the widespread interfaith services throughout the country, reinforced an accurate, undeniable message about American culture: grief unites us. The same article mentioned that debris from the World Trade Center—the material remains of decimated buildings and annihilated bodies mixed together into sacred ruins—had been transported to cities throughout the nation for ritual purposes. In San Clemente, California, for example, "surfers in a competition were to paddle into a circle and sprinkle Ground Zero dust in the Pacific Ocean." A monument that included "hundreds of pounds of contorted metal from Ground Zero" was unveiled in Eastlake, Ohio.[11]

Numerous stories appeared in the media about Ground Zero as holy ground that could not be contained at the site, nor kept from Americans who felt emotionally and spiritually attached to dirt and rocks that remained where the Twin Towers once stood. For example, the *New York Post* covered the anniversary ceremonies there in an article headlined "Even dirt is hallowed as loved ones collect scraps of memories," on September 12, 2002. The story begins, "They brought their grief and love, and they left with a handful of stones, a bag of dirt or a scrap of metal." The writers then recount how many individuals attending the ceremony at Ground Zero removed "hallowed earth of the World Trade Center site" for deeply personal reasons tied to memory, identity, and material reminders of what has been lost under these horrible conditions, forcing humans to confront a particularly cruel dilemma for grief: no bodies.[12] Ongoing public focus on this dilemma, reflected in but also shaped by media coverage, made sure the sites of destruction were not devoid of the sacred or without the possibility of some form of redemption.

In another example of how a killing field was translated into sacred ground that simultaneously remains in New York and can be transportable to other parts of the country, the *Dallas Morning News* reported on the design proposal for Texas' 9/11 memorial. The granite and steel monument will incorporate beams from the rubble at Ground Zero and have engravings that will remind visitors of a nation's commitment to the dead, including "Peace and Freedom Will Prevail" and "We Will Not Falter." The design architect is quoted as saying: "We want people to feel the relics that were washed in the blood of innocents. We want people to recognize the horror, understand the sorrow, the righteous wrath, the resolve and remembrance."[13]

Although ritual acts, public speeches, and individual comments attempting to make sense of the shock and sorrow associated with 9/11 varied throughout the nation, media reports celebrated the unified determination of the entire country to keep the dead in mind, and to be reconciled to their disturbing, yet inspiring, presence in the collective imagination. The tone of most stories that called attention to the sacrifice of the dead was respectful and honorable, a fitting attempt to bring dignity to the thousands of people who died by linking their fate to the fate of the nation.

In Don Collins's story for CBSNews.com on September 11, 2002, the loss of a strong, widespread national "connectedness" which materialized in the weeks and months after the attacks could be recovered by the public focus on the dead a year after the fact: "Hundreds of ceremonies around the country will mark the first anniversary of the disaster. These gatherings will honor the dead, but they can also be seen as an effort to rekindle at least a part of the magical spirit that brought the country so closely together in the days, weeks and months following the attacks."[14] National unity and spiritual invigoration are tied specifically to remembering the dead, identifying with them as heroic Americans whose deaths speak to numerous individual lives cut short but also to common cause and collective renewal.

In a September 13 *USA Today* piece entitled "Coverage of 9/11/02 was hard to criticize," Peter Johnson quotes academics and anchors from national news outlets as being quite satisfied with how media handled the coverage on the anniversary generally, and how the public spotlight on the dead evoked feelings of national pride more specifically. While some considered the coverage excessive, Brit Hume holds up the broadcast and cable network airing of the roll calls of names of the deceased as particularly revealing of national character: "It showed our reverence for life, which distinguishes us from the people who acted against us and consider life cheap and expendable."[15]

In spite of the lingering feeling that this day was unparalleled in American history, news reports included various efforts to think about 9/11 in familiar and time-tested terms. The *Houston Chronicle*, for example, quotes Virginia Van Cleave, president of the Daughters of the Republic of Texas, in the article: "For a day, we were all as one." She placed the dead from 9/11 into a well-known mythological landscape at one of the nation's most revered sites in the southwest, the Alamo: "How appropriate it is that we should be conducting this commemoration at a place where another group of common people made the ultimate sacrifice for freedom."[16] Journalists also mentioned the attack on Pearl Harbor as well as the more recent tragedy at the Murrah building in Oklahoma City. One year after the event, public culture provided many Americans with frames of reference with which to put the memory of the 9/11 dead in an appropriate imaginative, but historically scripted, context.

This rhetorical effort to transform innocent, unsuspecting civilians into national heroes who sacrificed their lives—often implicitly compared to American soldiers who died fighting for the country in wars past—is a popular strategy to reassure American citizens that these deaths were not meaningless, and that American justice will prevail. In Los Angeles, the *Daily News* published an editorial entitled "Uniting America; Renewing the National Resolve" the day after the first-year anniversary. It begins: "The nation grieved Wednesday for the 3,025 innocent victims of the Sept. 11 terrorist attacks, and today marks an anniversary of another sort. It was on this day a year ago . . . that we steeled ourselves with a new sense of resolve, a resolve to defeat our enemies and prevent another atrocity. As we mark that anniversary, we must renew that resolve."[17] It then reiterates many of the explicit and implicit messages communicated by President Bush during the day of national mourning: the dead will be avenged, and the nation will ultimately triumph over evil terrorists.

President Bush and his speechwriters understood the vital links between the body politic and the blood of martyrs, a strikingly religious theme echoed throughout American history generally, but most powerfully articulated by Abraham Lincoln in the Gettysburg Address—a sacred text recited during the memorial services in New York City. In the president's remarks at the Pentagon, for example, the 9/11 dead were front and center as inspirational touchstones for the continuing war on terrorism in general and the invasion of Afghanistan in particular: "Their loss has moved a nation to action, in a cause to defend other innocent lives in the world. . . . In every turn of this war, we will always remember how it began, and who fell first."[18] And later in the day at Ellis Island, after musing philosophically about the shortness of our days here on earth, he emphasized the same political, and deeply religious, point about these inspiring martyrs: "We resolved a year ago to honor every last person lost. We owe them remembrance and we owe them more. We owe them, and their children, and our own, the most enduring monument we can build: a world of liberty and security made possible by the way America leads."[19]

Very few people called into question Bush's remarks and the public acts memorializing 9/11 after the one-year anniversary. But some raised questions about Bush's policies and the political uses of the dead from this tragic day. On September 19, 2002, politics professor Bradley Gitz wondered in an editorial for the *Arkansas Democrat-Gazette* whether he was "the only one who found last week's commemoration of Sept. 11 a wee bit excessive and syrupy, perhaps driven a tad too much by television melodrama and choreographed sentiment?"[20] For the higher-profile Michael Kinsley in the September 20, 2002, *Washington Post*, the knee-jerk reliance on a simplistic worldview of good versus evil was an inappropriate response in the wake of such an act of terror: "There are many groups of people, unfortunately, who would be happy to hijack four airplanes, fly them into crowded buildings and kill 3,000 Americans. In terms of malign intent, they are all evil. But only one of them managed to do it. The concept of evil tells you nothing about why—among the many evils wished upon the United States—this one actually happened. Nor does 'evil' help us figure out how to stop evil from visiting itself upon us again."[21]

Whether Bush is portrayed as emotionally soft or conceptually limited, his presidential words about the enduring monument—a world of liberty and security—owed to the dead is defining his legacy in U.S. history. From the war in Afghanistan to the war against Iraq, President Bush's authority and presidential standing is based, for many Americans, in large part on his response to the dead and the foreign and domestic policy changes that have resulted from September 11, 2001.

Is this really what the living owe the dead in the wake of 9/11? Do we all agree about the role of these victims in national life generally, and military strategy particularly? Contrary to conventional wisdom about America as the epitome of a death-denying culture, U.S. history is riddled with examples of obsessive interest in, if not downright cultic activity surrounding, the bones of the dead. The history of death in America is full of conflict as well as consensus, division as much as solidarity. Think of the widespread pillaging of Native America graves, the urgent politicizing of the Civil War dead (on both sides), the divisive quarrelling over the questionable sacrifices in Vietnam—in addition to the ongoing efforts to recover the remains of soldiers missing in action, to name only a few examples.

America has always relied on the dead to define itself and its mission in the world. For Bush and numerous journalists who are attuned to the value of promoting a vision of social unity and common cause, our understandings of and interactions with these dead bind us together and reflect national commitments to act appropriately in the face of these atrocities. But the contestations over the meaning of the dead—a recurring symbolic struggle with profoundly high stakes, especially in times of crisis—suggest that automatic assumptions about collective solidarity often gloss over real divisions. For example, many of those who lost a loved one on that day have banded together to publicly declare their opposition to the war with Iraq. For these survivors, war is not the answer and will not bring dignity to the deaths of their family members and friends. One recent bumper sticker reads "Our Grief Is Not a Declaration of War," a stark and disturbing challenge to the unquestioned appropriation of the dead to prop up the war machine. The conflict over how to live with this grief has yet to be resolved, and what actions can salve the deeply traumatic memories of that day of death and destruction are yet to be determined.

Final Thoughts

In the weeks, months, and years after 9/11, Americans have grappled with the ultimate meaning of the dead and their destiny on the cultural landscape—both the physical, material landscapes devoted to monuments that memorialize, and the symbolic, spiritual landscapes devoted to memories that give their lives, and deaths, monumental meaning. Public culture is a crucial arena where these negotiations over the proper meaning of the dead and vitality of civil religion are worked out. In the case of the 9/11 victims, whose deaths could not be easily associated with time-tested scripts to make sense of the carnage of that day, a combination of formal and informal ritual strategies, popular expressions of sorrow and transcendence, and efforts to tie their sacrifices to national identity were used to reconcile the living with the dead.

All three cultural moments explored above—the immediate aftermath of the terrorist strike, the release and reception of Bruce Springsteen's latest album, and the media coverage of the one-year anniversary commemorations around the country—gave new life to the memory of those individuals who died on September 11, 2001. The news from that day and the images seared into our personal and popular consciousness conveyed the kind of horror generally reserved for big-budget Hollywood blockbusters celebrating awe-inspiring technical effects that promise spectacular violence and extraordinary destruction without real bodies to bury. Many Americans remarked that what they were seeing reminded them of a film-going experience.

But the real trauma to the national psyche and the shared mourning experienced in the wake of the destruction called for shared interpretations of these deaths and nationally sanctioned efforts to ritually incorporate the dead into the hearts and minds of the living. The American public could not understand those who perished from the attacks as dying in vain, or without meaning, or, worse still, only with the meanings determined by their killers. The circumstances of their deaths, the obliteration of their bodies, and the symbolic potency of the targets made the cultural work of reconciliation with these deaths an especially delicate task for a public that immediately recognized the challenges of living with them for a long time to come.

Notes

1. Somini Sengupta, "Rites of Grief, Without a Body to Cry Over," *The New York Times* (September 27, 2001): E1.

2. Margaret Woodbury, "With Bodies Lost in the Rubble, Mourners Forgo Traditional Rites," *San Francisco Chronicle* (October 14, 2001): 1.

3. Dean E. Murphy, "Slowly, Families Accept the Ruins as Burial Ground," *The New York Times* (September 29, 2001): 1.

4. Jane Spencer and Jennifer Tanaka, "Final Respects: New York's Funeral Industry Prepares for an Onslaught," *Newsweek*, September 22, 2001. Available at: www.msnbc.com.news/632663.asp (September 25, 2002).

5. No author, "The *New York Times* 'Portraits of Grief,'" CBSNews.com, September 11, 2002. Available at: www.cbsnews.com/stories/2002/09/10/earlyshow/leisure/books/printable521377.shtml (September 28, 2002).

6. Janny Scott, "A Nation Challenged: The Portraits; Closing a Scrapbook Full of Life and Sorrow," *The New York Times* (December 31, 2001): B6.

7. David Browne, "Review: Springsteen Relevant in 'Rising,'" CNN.com, July 29, 2002. Available at: www.cnn.com/2002/SHOWBIZ/Music/07/29/ew.rec.mus.rising (February 12, 2003).

8. Gregory Heisler, "Bruce Rising," *Time* (August 5, 2002): 56.

9. Richard Vara and Tara Dooley, "Thousands Crowd Places of Worship to Find Solace," *Houston Chronicle*, September 12, 2002. Available at: www.chron.com/CDA/story.hts/special/sept11/1571572 (July 2, 2003).

10. Phil Fairbanks, "A Call to Remember," *Buffalo News* (September 12, 2002): 1.

11. "Americans Remember 9/11 in Many Different Ways," CNN.com, September 11, 2002. Available at: www.cnn.com/2002/US/09/11/ar911.memorial. nation (February 19, 2003).

12. Jeane MacIntosh and Bridget Harrison, "Even Dirt Is Hallowed as Loved Ones Collect Scraps of Memories," *New York Post*, September 12, 2002. Available at: www.nypost.com/09112002/56902.htm (March 1, 2003).

13. Christy Hoppe, "State's Sept. 11 Memorial: 'You Feel It in Your Soul," *Dal-*

las Morning News, September 12, 2002. Available at: www.dallasnews.com/sharedcontent/dallas/nation/9-11/stories/091202dntextxmemorial.3b05.html (July 2, 2003).

14. Dan Collins, "September 11: One Year Later," CBSNews.com, September 9, 2002. Available at: www.cbsnews.com/stories/2002/09/04/september11/main520816.shtml (February 2, 2003).

15. Peter Johnson, "Coverage of 9/11/02 Was Hard to Criticize," *USA Today* (September 13, 2002): 1.

16. Alan Bernstein, "For a Day, We Were All as One," *Houston Chronicle*, September 12, 2002. Available at: www.cbsnews.com/stories/2002/09/04/september11/main520816.shtml (July 2, 2003).

17. Editorial, "Uniting America; Renewing the National Resolve," *The Daily News* (September 12, 2002): C4.

18. President George W. Bush's Remarks at the Pentagon, CNN.com, September 11, 2002. Available at: www.cnn.com/2002/US/09/11/ar911.bush.pentagon (July 2, 2003).

19. President George W. Bush's Remarks at Ellis Island, September 11, 2002. Available at: www.whitehouse.gov/news/releases/2002/09/20020911-3.html (July 2, 2003).

20. Bradley Gitz, "Editorial," *Arkansas Democrat-Gazette* (September 19, 2002): 14.

21. Michael Kinsley, "Deliver Us from Evil," *Washington Post*, September 20, 2002. Available at: www.washingtonpost.com/ac2/wp-dyn/A42099-2002Sep19 (February 23, 2002).

Vengeance Is Never Enough

Alternative Visions of Justice

Theophus Smith

In this essay I address why vengeance is never enough. More specifically, I explore why we "can't get no satisfaction" from retributive justice—the typical system of justice based on retaliation for crime. The September 11th terrorist attacks on the United States offer a point of departure for framing the issue of retributive justice versus an alternative —restorative justice.[1] Restorative justice seeks the restoration of just relationships between conflicted parties. A clearer perspective on that topic may be gained through examining a case study that explores the moral and therapeutic merits of a restorative justice approach. This case study involves lawsuits filed by native people in Canada who were abused in residential schools as children. The schools were operated not only by the government but also by various churches. I focus in particular on the Anglican Church of Canada and the pivotal nature of shame in ongoing conflicts. That case illuminates the resolution of and connections among the shame experienced by victims, perpetrators, and collective groups in national contexts.

The days following September 11, 2001, provided an opportunity far more unique than the events of September 11 itself.[2] For the first time, the possibility arose for establishing restorative justice on a global scale. Restorative justice, in contrast to conventional forms of retaliation or retributive justice, seeks to rectify not only violations of law perpetrated by offenders against their victims, but also the larger social relations that are impaired by such violations.[3] Hoping against hope for such a possibility, communities across the world waited in the days immediately following the terrorist attacks to see how the new president of the world's only remaining superpower would deal with such a massive as-

35

sault. Would conventional acts of retaliation ensue—"retributive justice" in the terms discussed in this essay? Or would a heretofore unseen order of statesmanship emerge, something comparable to Nelson Mandela's leadership in fostering South Africa's Truth and Reconciliation Commission in the mid-1990s?

What was possible in those weeks while the world waited was the postponing of military force for just long enough (perhaps indefinitely) to achieve something else instead: something that would set a precedent in the new millennium for how a world power deals with a major threat to its own security and to global stability, something that would render the world safer from terrorist threats than any resort to mere war could ever achieve.

Instead, our nation's collective mortification and shame led to a policy of retaliation motivated by the need to "cover up" our own national security misjudgments: the errors of our government, of our intelligence agencies, and of our military institutions. By focusing attention on vengeance against enemies, a novice administration diverted attention from our national state of unpreparedness, inattention to foreign affairs, and the resulting failure to foresee and forestall the September 11th attacks. The following case study explores in more detail the nature of such collective shame in relation to retributive justice on the one hand, and restorative justice on the other.

Collective Shame: The Case of the Anglican Church of Canada

The Anglican Church of Canada is currently undergoing an excruciating time as part of a national trauma that at one point threatened to bankrupt the church. It involves a history of sex crimes in which both church and state were complicit, and it raises all the issues of restorative justice that concern us here. The tragic story begins in the early nineteenth century, when the Canadian government developed and carried out a federal policy of assimilating the country's indigenous peoples into mainstream society. The explicit goal was to eradicate what was termed the "Indian problem" by changing "first nations" peoples into conventional Canadian citizens. The result, however, was a brutal attack on native cultures, the effects of which continue today in communities struggling with alcohol and drug addiction, suicide and sexual abuse, and a host of other family and social disorders.

One of the most traumatizing outcomes of this policy occurred in the residential schools for those called "Indians." These schools were operated not only by the government but also by Christian churches. Specifically, four churches ran approximately 130 residential schools for native children, stretching across the continent from Vancouver Island in the west to Nova Scotia in the east. These were run by Anglican, Roman Catholic, Presbyterian, and Methodist churches. About 105,000 children across the country attended these church schools, among whom some 35,000 attended the 28 schools operated by Anglican churches. Altogether, Anglican involvement in residential schools spanned 150 years, from the opening of the first school in 1820 to the closing of the last school in 1971.

Today many of these schools are a cause for national shame because of the epidemic levels of sexual abuse that occurred in them, lasting up until that last school closing in the early 1970s. According to David Napier,

> For the last few years, former attendees of residential schools have been coming forward in droves, claiming they were physically, sexually and mentally abused while students at these mostly remote schools that operated in Canada for more than a century. Thousands have retained lawyers and turned Canada's justice system into the backdrop for the ultimate national story of crime and punishment.[4]

By fall of 2002 some 12,000 of the 90,000 former students had filed claims against government-owned schools that were operated by the Anglican, Roman Catholic, Presbyterian, and United churches.[5] In the several hundred cases citing the Anglican Church as co-defendant, the suits named not only various dioceses (or church regions) but also the national church or General Synod, which had established the missionary society that ran most of the schools. The prospect of financial bankruptcy was imminent not only for those separate dioceses but also for the General Synod itself, which had assets of about $10 million, whereas the damages for which it might be liable were already exceeding $2 billion. Indeed, the thousands of former school attendees who were retaining lawyers made financial claims anticipated in the tens of billions of dollars.

In November 2002 the Anglican Church of Canada agreed to share the costs of the lawsuits with the Canadian government. Anglicans were implicated in some 18 percent of the cases whereas Roman Catholics were named in 73 percent; the United Church was implicated in 8 percent and Presbyterians in 1 percent. At this point only the Anglicans are included in the agreement with the government. According to the agreement, the Anglican Church would contribute up to $16 million (U.S. dollars) while the government would pay the rest of the total costs anticipated at $1 billion (Canadian dollars).[6]

In addition to such huge financial costs, the litigation had begun fracturing Canadian society. Native Anglicans have been pitted against the Anglican Church of Canada, and the church against the federal government. Take, for example, the first case to come to trial involving the Anglican Church, that of Floyd Mowatt, Sr., versus Derek Clarke. Clarke was Mowatt's dormitory supervisor between 1970 and 1973, beginning when Mowatt was nine years old. In 1999, Justice Janice Dillon found Clarke guilty of being a sexual predator in the eight years that he worked at the school, abusing children weekly and often daily. Then she assigned 60 percent of the share of liability to the Anglican Church and 40 percent to the Canadian government. But there are costs more grievous than disputing and sharing the burden of financial liability.

In Lytton, British Columbia, the site of St. George's Indian Residential School where Mowatt was a student, eight native men killed themselves the summer they received subpoenas as witnesses in that case. "Handing out those papers was one of the biggest mistakes the government ever made," one fellow survivor from St. George's observed. "They knew their secret was out. They thought, 'Everybody's gonna know that I let this guy do it to me for candy. . . . They were some of the toughest guys in town."[7] Obviously the most traumatic effects of litigation occurred among the survivors themselves, in ways that compounded their former victimization. It might have been anticipated that some of them would take their own lives rather than face the shame of having their secret victimization exposed in public trials in which they were called to appear as witnesses or co-plaintiffs. It is this dimension of shame that the adversarial court system can neither fathom nor adequately address. To navigate and negotiate that abyss of shame, one needs a system of restorative justice, not retributive justice.

But in addition to the shame associated with the act of being abused, there is another level of shame that attaches to the cash settlements awarded in such cases. Said one survivor: "Around here it's called 'arse money.' It's supposed to be dirty." But this particular survivor has done enough of his own healing work to acknowledge that, as he surmised, "such taunts often come from people who have suffered abuse them-selves and are simply hiding behind catcalls rather than face their own demons."[8] In any case, "many victims who've gone the legal route feel cheated—even after they win in court."[9]

In this connection, the issue of victim compensation or "satisfaction" becomes key.

> [First nations'] traditions dictate that justice be meted out in the form of shame rather than physical punishment or incarceration . . . [they] are often uncomfortable seeking retribution within a European-based justice system. . . . Only a small degree of *satisfaction* comes from squaring off against an abuser—something few plaintiffs get to do anyway, given that defendants are usually represented by legal counsel and not required to appear in court. [Emphasis mine.]

Elaborating on this issue of "satisfaction," Dr. Maggie Hodgson, head of the Assembly of First Nations' alternative dispute resolution team, acknowledged that "There ain't a hell of a lot that's right with litigation. . . . At no place does it spell humanity." In a related comment, Russell Raikes, a lawyer in London, Ontario, whose clients include hundreds of claimants, observed that "Right now [year 2000] there's only one place to resolve these issues, and that's in court. Until there's another option, or they invent a better mousetrap, that's the way to go."[10]

Here I conclude our brief case study by following Attorney Raikes's reference to finding "another option" or, as he also says, inventing "a better mousetrap." But I propose a "mousetrap" not for snaring sexual predators, or for exposing and pillorying church and state for their joint complicity in a national shame. Rather I propose a "trap" for capturing and harnessing shame itself. For, as recent studies indicate, shame is the key dynamic that operates in and motivates retributive justice. On the basis of such studies I hypothesize that managing shame is the central issue in converting our justice systems from retributive values to restor-ative values.

And here I refer not simply to the shame of the victim, but also to the shame of the perpetrator. Nor does our shame analysis end there. Finally, we must face our collective, communal shame as the commu-nity in which such behaviors occur. That is the unspoken shame that we all harbor as part of a public in which we either know, have known, or could know—if we were making it our business to pay attention—such perpetrators and such victims. It includes the shame of our own potential, if not actual, complicity in institutions, organizations, interest groups, and family systems that enable or permit such victims and their perpetrators to exist.

From the perspective of this kind of shame analysis, we all need restoration on the other side of injustice and abuse. Indeed, one of the holistic goals of restorative justice is the restoration of the community itself. For the community, on the one hand, is also included among the parties who have been offended and violated alongside the victim. And on the other hand, the community is situated alongside the offender as well, insofar as we all have an uneasy conscience that "we have left undone those things which we ought to have done, and we have done those things which we ought not to have done," as the prayer of "Confession" puts it in the Episcopal Church's prayer book.[11]

Toward a Unified Theory in Ethics and Psychology, Law and Religion[12]

In this segment I turn to the results of a convergent effort to explore the requirements of restorative justice. I refer to the research and scholarship of sociologist Thomas Scheff, professor emeritus of the University of California at Santa Barbara, and his wife Suzanne Retzinger. Beginning in the 1990s with their book *Emotions and Violence: Shame and Rage in Destructive Conflicts*, Scheff and Retzinger have been pioneers in studying the relationship of shame management and anger management to alternative approaches in the criminal justice system.[13] In a report on their research first published in the University of Puerto Rico law journal *Revista Jurídica*, Scheff attempted to advance the development of restorative justice by means of insights from the field of "therapeutic jurisprudence."[14] Taking together the fields of restorative justice and therapeutic jurisprudence, Scheff combined them in a single expression that he called "RTJ." He then justified that compound expression in the following terms:

> In recent years, an alternative approach to law, a worldwide movement, has been building momentum. This movement has two vectors, restorative justice and therapeutic jurisprudence (RTJ). RTJ has the potential to resolve many kinds of conflict and reduce inequities in the legal system. Compared to the traditional legal model of justice, courts, judges, lawyers and prisons, restorative justice and therapeutic jurisprudence are quite similar. The difference between the two is mostly conceptual. As a frame within which to criticize and modify legal justice, therapeutic jurispru-

dence offers a strikingly different model, the mode of therapy as it is used in medical and psychological treatment. Although close inspection reveals that the therapeutic model is quite diverse, and therefore somewhat ambiguous, it does offer a framework to contrast with the legal model. Although restorative justice is the larger movement of the two, it suffers from the lack of such a model. Without a model, restorative justice offers piecemeal changes to correct the present legal system. Perhaps a welding together of the two models into one, RTJ, would make the movement more effective.[15]

The linchpin of Scheff's effort to combine the two models comes out of the mediation movement, and specifically a form of victim–offender mediation called "community conferencing." Such conferences divert the offender from the courtroom into an alternative system. Also known as "family group conferencing," this alternative creates a meeting between the victim, the offender, and other parties interested in a resolution of the case. Since the late 1980s, when a conferencing law was passed in New Zealand, community conferences have become the most developed form of victim–offender mediation. In Australia conferencing has been used for both juvenile and adult crimes, and the format has also been applied in certain cities in the United States and England.

The conference format typically involves four steps. First, the offender describes his or her own offense in detail. Next, the facilitator asks the offender to describe the consequences of the offense, how it affected him, and how it affected the victim and others. Third, the victim and the victim's supporters tell how the crime affected them. This step is often highly emotional, with visible tears and/or anger. The last part of the conference entails working out a settlement that is acceptable to both victim and offender.

Now, as Scheff goes on to emphasize, if this emotional part of the conference is managed successfully, then the new procedure has a powerful advantage over the conventional courtroom process. Its obvious advantage is that it allows direct communication between offenders and their victims. With such immediacy the possibility arises, on the one hand, of a larger community involvement in the process. On the other hand, and partly due to this expanded involvement, the possibility also arises of negotiation and understanding, contrition and confession, reconciliation and forgiveness. Scheff aggregates these features under the term "symbolic reparation," by which he refers (more precisely) to the emotional preconditions for "repairing" the relationship between victim and offender. Those preconditions are quite familiar and obvious, but often arduous to achieve: respect and courtesy, regret or remorse, apology and forgiveness. They constitute the very elements that are ruled out by the conventional court system precisely because it structurally avoids direct communication between offender and victim. And since the more substantive forms of material reparation—that is, the actual settlement—are so much easier to negotiate when such emotional reparation occurs, the management of emotional processes becomes a crucial factor in therapeutic jurisprudence and in RTJ.

Emotional reparation (my preferred term here) as understood by Scheff involves social rituals of respect, courtesy, apology, and forgiveness that can operate independently of verbal discourse and that depend on the emotional dynamics of the parties involved in the meeting. In particular, the emotions of shame and anger are key, including the management of moral indignation as it arises in the victim and among other participants. In this regard, Scheff has identified two steps in what he calls the "core sequence" of achieving emotional reparation. First, the offender must clearly express genuine shame and remorse regarding the offenses committed. Only then can the second step of genuine forgiveness be managed by the victim and the victim's community—genuine because it occurs without coercion or pressure from the facilitator or the community.

With this two-step core sequence, which may take only a few seconds, the basis is laid for a more extensive step: the offender's reintegration into the community with less likelihood of becoming a stigmatized and therefore repeat offender. Moreover, with such "emotional conciliation," Scheff insists, the actual settlement of the case is more likely to satisfy all the participants by being neither too lenient nor too punitive. Without the core sequence, any material settlement typically leaves the parties instead with a high level of unreleased tension, and with a feeling of the arbitrariness of the settlement and a persistent or recurrent sense of dissatisfaction. In fact, apart from the elements of emotional reparation, all the innovations discussed so far (from community conferencing to the larger mediation movement, and from therapeutic jurisprudence to RTJ generally) may in the final analysis result in only superficial alternatives to conventional courtroom practices. For, Scheff claims, emotional reparation is the key criterion that distinguishes conferencing from its predecessor forms of criminal justice.

Restorative Justice and the Transformation of Shaming

Now let's take a look at the management of shame, anger, and moral indignation in therapeutic jurisprudence. A key feature in this connection is what Scheff calls "reintegrative shaming," borrowing the expression from John Braithwaite in his book on *Crime, Shame and Reintegration*.[16] For reintegration of an offender to occur following conviction and sentencing, Braithwaite determines, the process must achieve the following balance: enough shaming for the seriousness of the offense to be made clear, but not so much that the level of humiliation plunges the offender into hopelessness, bitterness, and spitefulness toward rejoining the community.

A persuasive example comes from English history when the punishment for theft was being branded with a hot iron on one's forehead with the letter "F"—that is, for felon. Not surprisingly, this "cruel and unusual" practice actually increased the incidence of the crime, since branded persons were so conspicuously excluded from normal society that they had no recourse but to seek the company of a criminal community. Too much offender shame, Scheff concludes, can be just as destructive for the larger community as too little.

The balance that community conferences seek consists in transferring all the shame connected to the crime from the victim to the offender, but without the surplus shaming that derives from the victim's and the community's unprocessed anger and moral indignation. The first stage of this transferring process is key. The victim must be relieved of humiliation deriving from the degradation, betrayal, and violation that has been inflicted by the offense. Conventional court procedures actually do little to achieve this relief, Scheff points out. He then goes on to suggest that such leftover humiliation in the courtroom may drive the victim and the larger public to seek excessive punishment of the offender. Surplus shaming thus appears as a crude and unreflective effort to get the emotional compensation that the justice system fails to provide in a normative and structural manner.

But the second stage in shame management is also key. The purpose for the offender's accepting all of the shame connected to the offense is so that he or she may take the next step toward facing the victim and offering the signs of emotional reparation. Only such a step has a chance of relieving the victim of his or her emotional suffering. For the facilitator's restraint in transferring shame from the victim to the offender is not only for the sake of the offender's reintegration into the community following the conference. It is also necessary for the sake of the victim during the conference itself. Only by means of such restraint will the offender be left with sufficient dignity or humanity intact to be able to show the impact of the transferred shame. Otherwise an emotional constriction or hardening occurs, attended by the kind of denial of accountability that we have all experienced when the impact (or prospect) of shame and humiliation seems too great to endure.[17]

Instead of denial, it is the showing of the offender's shame to the victim and to the observing community that is transformative. The reason for this transformation is twofold. On the one hand, the fact that one's offender shows visible shame for his or her misconduct is transformative for the victim. For this visible fact helps transfer or dissolve the victim's sense of shame, humiliation, and violation—thus repairing or restoring the victim's humanity. On the other hand, showing some degree of visible shame can be transformative for the offender because it also restores or repairs his or her humanity. However, it remains key, to reiterate, that the offender not be induced to experience excessive shame in violation of his or her humanity, which is precisely the prospect that offenders find so forbidding that they eschew showing visible shame altogether, preferring denial of their misconduct or avoidance of courtroom encounters with their victims. Admittedly, it requires uncommonly humane skill and care for the offender to be granted an opportunity to show visible shame without too great a risk of incurring excess shame.

In any case, Scheff remarks:

> The offender must be ashamed of what he did, and this shame must be visible to the [victim/community]. It is this shame—along with other emotions, such as grief—that allows a preliminary bond to be formed between offender and victim, because the offender's visible expression of emotion allows the victim to see the offender as a human being.[18]

With this formulation we arrive at the crucial determining factor in community conferencing, therapeutic jurisprudence, and restorative justice or RTJ generally. The crucial factor resides in the capacity of the practices involved to restore or repair the co-humanity of both victim and offender in the context of a skilled and enabling community. Such a community is mature enough, in Scheff's words, "to manage shame beneficially . . . to recover the positive, reconciliatory uses of normal shame from the maws of repression and silence, and to relearn its value as a powerful emotion for forming community."[19] Such a community is also mature enough, he goes on to show, to help the victim and other participants to manage their anger and moral indignation as well as their shame.

> The crucial point about moral indignation is that when it is repetitive and out of control, it is a defensive movement. It involves two steps: denial of one's own shame, followed by projection of blame onto the offender (I am not dishonorable in any way, whereas the offender is entirely dishonorable). For the participants to identify with the offender, they must see themselves as alike rather than unalike (there but for the grace of God go I). . . . Thus, uncontrolled, repetitive moral indignation is the most important impediment to symbolic reparation and reintegration. On the other hand, to the extent that it is rechanneled, moral indignation can be instrumental in triggering the core sequence of reparation.[20]

Such skillful management of moral indignation offers an additional challenge in the management of shame. Scheff's claim that moral indignation must be "rechanneled" requires integrating indignation within a larger purpose: that of transforming (or restoring) victim–offender relations. Since excess or repetitive indignation is an "impediment" to such transformation, a more instrumental or mediating use of indignation must be found. The key to this instrumentality resides in what Scheff describes as identification with the offender: "participants . . . must see themselves as alike rather than unalike (there but for the grace of God go I)." To the contrary, runaway moral indignation constitutes a projection of surplus blame onto offenders: "I am not dishonorable in any way, whereas you are entirely dishonorable"; or "even under similar circumstances I would never act as despicably as you have." In effect this attitude denies our co-humanity with offenders.

As if attempting to reinstate that co-humanity, however, offenders typically resist admitting their moral accountability in the face of our runaway indignation. For they intrinsically understand that their crimes or misdeeds were sometimes passively and even actively supported or abetted by dysfunctional and vicious institutions and systems in the larger society. They rightly intuit that they are being targeted with a surplus of blame when the community singles them out, exclusively, for actions that in fact characterize anti-social practices prevailing elsewhere in society. A society's inability to take account of its own dysfunctions, as a contributing factor in the misdeeds of its offenders, constitutes scapegoating offenders for activities that it is not mature enough to face *en masse* or at large. A more mature and anti-scapegoating ethic consists, by contrast, in summoning all parties to acknowledge and value the co-humanity of offenders.

To admit this co-humanity is not to exonerate offenders' crimes or misdeeds, but rather to mediate the process by which they may be induced to offer "symbolic reparation" (Scheff). As introduced above, symbolic reparation involves social expressions of respect and courtesy, regret or remorse, apology and forgiveness. In this regard it often precedes, and enables offenders to agree to, material reparation. Thus, acknowledging offenders' co-humanity can establish an ethic of reciprocity: a moral basis for acknowledging and symbolically restoring the violated humanity of their victims.

Restorative Justice Following September 11

But what if offenders are constitutionally incapable of rendering reparations, either symbolic or material? What if no sensibilities of human reciprocity can be established as a basis for moral appeal? What if neither our offenders, nor indeed ourselves, are inclined to acknowledge our co-humanity in any substantive way? That appears to be the situation as regards the United States and its terrorist enemies following September 11, 2001. On its basis the most banal expressions of moral indignation became popular in the United States, and the most conventional forms of retributive justice became dominant in pursuit of a military solution to the crisis of global terrorism. Is there any alternative, particularly in view of our discussion above regarding shame management as a key constituent of restorative justice?

The following alternative is based on this foundational insight of restorative justice: that we are all longing for our respective communities to find ways to restore our dignity and worth even (especially) after our most traumatizing and shame-filled experiences of violation. In the context of September 11, this perennial human longing can be addressed in the following way.

In the introduction to this essay I represented September 11 as the first time the possibility arose for establishing restorative justice on a global scale. What became available on that epochal day was the singular ability, rarely available to a nation-state, to define a new standard of civilization for all subsequent history: specifically, a new standard for the world order emerging after the fall of communism in the former Soviet Union. Such a geopolitical consensus was more likely immediately following September 11—on the corpses of the thousands of the dead, as it were. But the following alternative remains possible in the face of continuing terrorist crises worldwide. It remains possible, to be specific, to call for an international and inter-religious consensus establishing a new world standard: No killing of innocents is sanctioned by our nation or its religions.

There is no killing of innocents sanctioned by our nation or its religions. That claim is the single most contested principle of civilization (and civility) that remains to become normative in human history. To date, no nation and no religion (not even Buddhism) has been able to establish that standard in a way that is compelling and binding on all its adherents or leaders. Heretofore, rather, every tradition and every state has retained a belief in sacred violence: the belief in violence as the god of last resort who will save us when all else fails, the belief in violence "in the name of God" or in our own name—the name of the people or the state.

For the first time after September 11, a superpower was positioned with enough moral authority (and international sympathy for its victims) to call for a new standard in geopolitical relations. The United States was positioned, indeed, to call on heads of governments and key religious leaders of the world to: (1) reject the killing of innocents as a new standard in both civil and religious law, and thereby (2) make anti-terrorism a new standard in both civil and religious law. In particular, it was well positioned to challenge our Muslim allies here and abroad to join us in sanctions against the al-Qaeda network and the Taliban as *terrorist* entities and not as authentic *Muslim* societies.

Even now it remains possible for any nation or international organization to call on all world leaders, governmental bodies, and religious councils to rule publicly and unequivocally against the killing of innocent victims (so-called collateral damage) in the name of God or the state. In this way we would bring to the bar proponents of the major world religions and challenge them to disavow the exploitation and abuse of their traditions by terrorists who are pseudo-Muslim, pseudo-Jewish, and pseudo-Christian. Indeed, for many of our Muslim allies we would achieve from outside their countries what they themselves are not able to achieve internally: the long-awaited movement toward an Islam that is politically and ideologically moderate and that can restrain the more extremist, repressive, and entrenched representatives of that faith.

Such moral and enlightened leadership would empower Muslim moderates in relationship to their own political and religious leaders and in relation to their own peoples. And only such a consensus would render the world ultimately secure from terrorism, because only such a consensus can expose, disable, and disempower terrorism *from within* as a distorted form of extremist religion. Finally, only such a consensus can propagate a standard of civility and humanity among nations that the September 11th attacks attempted to preclude. It is appreciable, however, that we will continue to forfeit such new order statesmanship by pursuing military actions that incur the killing of innocents. Moreover, the shame-based motivation for such military actions will continue to give the lie to any claims of moral justification or arguments that distributive justice (compensating victims and punishing offenders) is the primary motivation involved.

Only a policy of moral restoration, not military reaction, can address the collective shame of our national unpreparedness for this new era of terrorism. The more mature and effective way to recover from such shame, as we have seen above, is to confront perpetrators within their own communities of accountability. The kind of community conferencing examined above suggests ways to do that—ways that can be extended, *by hypothesis*, to international and interfaith conflicts. More extensive consideration of such a hypothesis must await an essay specifically devoted to that concern (how to extrapolate, for example, from forms of restorative justice that address criminal justice to forms that address international and interfaith conflict.) But enough has been discovered here for us to answer the opening questions, why "vengeance is never enough"; and "why we 'can't get no satisfaction' from retributive justice.'"

Satisfaction eludes practitioners of retributive justice because such justice remains captive to the shame–rage cycle of injury-and-retaliation. What really satisfy, on the contrary, are procedures that enable us to resolve our shame in processes that simultaneously restore our humanity. Accordingly, we require processes that, at best, induce our perpetrators to offer symbolic reparations such as apologies, processes that restore to us the human dignity and worth wrested from us by their offenses. By contrast, reliance on victim compensation and offender punishment alone—that is, distributive justice—is insufficient to resolve issues of shame as experienced by some victims. Compensation as "shame money," for example, was the phenomenon described above in the case of some of the abuse survivors of Canadian residential schools. Other researchers offer the following explanation for the fact that victims may value apology as much as, or even more than, compensation.

> For some people, apology is more important than even rather generous financial compensation. Writing from a legal perspective, Hiroshi Wagatsuma and Arthur Rosett say that "there are some injuries that cannot be repaired just by saying you are sorry, and *there are others that can only be repaired by an apology.*" In the latter category are such injuries as *defamation, insult, degradation, and loss of status* [i.e., in my terms above, shame-based offenses]. All question the worth of a person. The message of worthlessness is taken back when the feelings and the moral status of the victim are acknowledged. . . . The explanation is to be found in the fact that *apology implies acknowledgement,* which can "unsay" the original message of insult.[21]

But if our perpetrators will not offer such forms of reparation, or cannot do so themselves, then their communities of accountability may be induced to do so on their behalf by cooperating with us through more creative and collective structures of restorative justice. The recent era of truth commissions augurs well for our ability to create such structures intra-nationally.[22] It remains to be seen whether we have the moral will and collective imagination to craft, and improve the effectiveness of, such restorative processes at the interfaith and geopolitical levels.

Notes

1. Retribution—that is, retaliation, revenge, or vengeance—contrasts with two other classic approaches to justice: the distributive and the restorative. Distributive justice is the proportional *distribution* of compensation to victims and punishment to perpetrators. Restorative justice, discussed in greater detail below, uses the framework of compensation and punishment as the means to a larger goal of *restoring* damaged relationships in the community where offenses occur by repairing where practicable the relationship between victims and offenders, and repairing as well the broader civic and social relationships that have been fractured by the offense.

2. On that day, terrorists using hijacked airplanes completed suicide flights that crashed into the World Trade Center in New York and the Pentagon in Washington, D.C., destroying the monolithic Twin Towers, killing nearly 3,000 people, and ushering in a new era of security vigilance for the United States and its Western allies.

3. Policies and programs that seek to "restore" relations between victims and their offenders, within the context of repairing an entire community, can include

restitution, memorials and civic events, public policy changes, and legal action resulting in either prosecution or conditional amnesty. South Africa's Truth and Reconciliation Commission (1995–98) is perhaps the most dramatic example.

4. David Napier, "Sins of the Fathers," *Anglican Journal* (May 2000): 2.

5. The United Church of Canada, which combined Methodist, Congregational, and some Presbyterian church bodies, was formed in 1925. For a history of the entity, see the United Church's website, www.united-church.ca/ucc/history.

6. James Solheim, Episcopal News Service, November 21, 2002.

7. Napier, "Sins of the Fathers," pp. 10–11.

8. Ibid., p. 7. In addition, this survivor "admits that dealing with lawyers and judges might not always be in his best interest, given that healing is what he craves, and this will not likely come via the adversarial court system."

9. Ibid., p. 12.

10. Ibid.

11. *The Book of Common Prayer* (New York: The Seabury Press, 1979), pp. 41–42.

12. My section title here anticipates the inclusion of religion in a unified theory of victim–perpetrator relations, but the scope of this essay does not permit me to develop that feature. Nonetheless I deem it important to retain the reference, particularly in view of the inclusion of an interfaith trajectory in the concluding section of this essay.

13. Thomas J. Scheff and Suzanne M. Retzinger, *Emotions and Violence: Shame and Rage in Destructive Conflicts* (Lexington, Mass.: Lexington Books, 1991). Cf. T.J. Scheff, *Catharsis in Healing, Ritual, and Drama* (Berkeley: University of California Press, 1979), 4.

14. *Revista Jurídica de la Universidad de Puerto Rico* (University of Puerto Rico, Rio Piedras Campus, School of Law) 59:1 (1990): 1–23.

15. Thomas J. Scheff, "Community Conferences: Shame and Anger in Therapeutic Jurisprudence," *Revista Jurídica* (U.P.R.) 59:1 (1990): 1–2.

16. John Braithwaite, *Crime, Shame and Reintegration* (New York: Cambridge University Press, 1989). Cf. John Braithwaite and Stephen Mugford, "Conditions of Successful Reintegration Ceremonies: Dealing with Juvenile Offenders," *The British Journal of Criminology* 34:2 (Spring 1994): 139–171.

17. In this regard we might attribute the protracted denials and public perjury of President Clinton during the 1998–99 investigation of his sex scandals to the forbidding prospect of the excess shaming that would also have ensued had he been truthful about his marital infidelities. If one accepts the logic that he had nothing to lose by lying—excess shaming would occur whether he lied or instead made an early admission of his culpability—then the emotional basis of his denial is obvious. This analysis does not address, of course, the normative issue of the president's moral resources, or the lack thereof, for facing the prospect of such shaming with courage and fortitude. Compare, in this connection (ironic?), the reference to President Clinton's official apology as head of state to Japanese Americans detained in camps during World War II, in note 21 below.

18. Scheff, "Community Conferences," p. 11.

19. Ibid., p. 10.

20. Ibid., p. 15.

21. Trudy Govier and Wilhelm Verwoerd, "The Promise and Pitfalls of Apolo-

gies," *Journal of Social Philosophy* 33:1 (Spring 2002), 71–72; the authors also quote Hiroshi Wagatsuma and Arthur Rosett in "The Implications of Apology: Law and Culture in Japan and the United States," *Law and Society Review*, no. 4 (1984) 461–98 (emphasis added). Consider President Clinton's 1998 apology to Japanese Americans, including government reparations, to redress their unconstitutional internment in detainee camps during World War II.

22. In the past twenty years the world has witnessed more than twenty truth commissions in places as disparate as Southeast Asia and South America. Perhaps most instructive for the United States are the commissions that have existed in South America and South Africa, notably:

Argentina's National Commission on Disappeared Persons (1984)
Chile's National Commission on Truth and Reconciliation (1991)
The United Nations Truth Commission for El Salvador (1993)
Guatemala's Commission for Historical Clarification (1996)
South Africa's Truth and Reconciliation Commission (1995–98).

Such exercises in "transitional justice" involve the efforts of "emerging democracies" to "cope with the legacy of an ousted repressive regime . . . [and] redress past abuses without creating new injustices, while peacefully integrating the victims and the perpetrators." Neil Kritz, *Transitional Justice: How Emerging Democracies Reckon with Former Regimes* (United States Institute of Peace, 1995).

More recently, new commissions have been operating or attempted in Bosnia-Herzegovina, the Federal Republic of Yugoslavia, East Timor, Nigeria, Panama, Sierra Leone, and Peru. Other countries are also considering convening truth commissions. In addition, various reparations programs have been established by governments around the world to assist the former victims of crimes committed by the state. In that connection the United Nations is involved in efforts to establish a set of universal principals on reparations to victims. (The International Center for Transitional Justice, 2001. Available at: www.ictj.org.)

Murder, Mourning, and the Ideal of Reconciliation

Tammy Krause

I wish I could take it back, but I can't. I'm so sorry. I wish there was a reason. There isn't. It's senseless. I wish I could point my finger at somebody else, anyone but myself, but I can't. I wish I didn't do what I did. . . . I wish Joie was here, but she's not. I wish I was not here, but I am. I have to face the reality of that. I'm sorry.[1]

—Cary Stayner, convicted of the murder of
Joie Armstrong, November 30, 2000

That was good because when he first started speaking, he was talking to the judge, and I thought, "We're the ones you should be talking to." He sounded sincere. He's devastated. . . . I ached for him. I ached for me. I ached for everything. . . . I will not live my life festering with anger, hatred, and vengeance. I won't do that.[2]

—Leslie Armstrong,
mother of Joie Armstrong, November 30, 2000

Reconciliation is not a goal in mind for families that have lost someone to homicide. For the Armstrong family, reconciliation was not a reason for the plea agreement they encouraged for Cary Stayner, who killed Joie Armstrong in Yosemite National Park. I met Joie's mother, Leslie Armstrong, in my role as a victim liaison—an intermediary who acts as a bridge between the surviving victim family members and the defense team.[3] The attorneys representing Cary Stayner asked if I would reach out to the Armstrong family with the goals of hearing the family's concerns surrounding Stayner's trial and to answer any questions they might have about the process.

Although relatively new within the legal system, the use of victim liaisons (also known as the practice of defense-based victim outreach) began in 1997 with the trial of Timothy McVeigh, the man convicted of the Oklahoma City bombing. McVeigh's attorneys became concerned about the impact a trial would have on the victim community and wanted to learn how they could best address their questions and concerns. This work is seen as controversial because it has been assumed that victims have no choice about their legal allegiance to the prosecution and that having any contact with the defense attorneys is inappropriate for both the defense attorneys and the victims' family members. Some defense attorneys, however, no longer accept relating to the victim survivors as a betrayal of the process or of their client, but rather as a way legal work should be done—both professionally and morally.

I have worked with many surviving family members since the McVeigh trial and have seen the enormous suffering they experience at the hands of the accused and the legal work done in the name of justice. After a murder, families are forced to deal with their grief in a public manner due to the judicial proceedings against the accused and the media's fascination with crime and death. The judicial system is a complex entity with which most citizens never interact. The system is even more difficult to understand when one is experiencing traumatic grief. To complicate matters, the judicial system is not designed to support the surviving family members due to its focus on the legal violations and actions of the defendant.

Because of this emphasis on the defense, families often feel revictimized by the judicial system, which ignores their concerns and needs. Defense-based victim outreach has shown the legal system that justice is far better served when victims' questions, concerns, and needs are formally addressed by the courts and, ultimately, by the defendant. I want to share stories of reconciliation in situations that seemed to offer no hope. The stories are not about the rare person able to rise above grief and vengeance—they are about ordinary citizens as flawed and human as I am. The decisions they made are remarkable considering the circumstances, but they will tell you that they were able to make certain choices because of the validation and support they were given by legal professionals.

This essay outlines several reasons that the concept of reconciliation seems implausible for surviving family members in homicide cases. While societal impediments often block reconciliation for survivors, there are steps that individuals, communities, and the legal system can take to remove these obstacles in surviving family members' journey of healing. Finally, this essay chronicles the turn of a few survivors toward reconciliation. Since so often the voice of the victims gets muddled in the clamor for justice, it is important to let their voices stand out on their own.

As I worked with the Armstrong family, they looked at the fact that although Stayner had confessed to killing Joie, a trial was inevitable and there would be years of court appeals because the federal government was seeking the death penalty against him. After we discussed the family's options and what their role would be in the judicial process, Joie's family decided to write a letter to the prosecutor trying the case against Cary Stayner. In the letter, they listed their needs and concerns in regards to the case against Stayner. They acknowledged that although there would be a certain satisfaction in seeing a jury sentence Stayner to death, more importantly, they wanted assurance that the judicial process would be final and no more money would be spent on his legal defense. Two months after the letter was written, Stayner changed his plea from not guilty to guilty and formally agreed to meet the concerns and conditions of the Armstrong family.

At the sentencing hearing, no one expected Cary Stayner to address Leslie Armstrong or Michael Raffaeli, Joie's fiancé. No one expected Ms. Armstrong to feel anguish for Stayner. It surprised everyone—journalists, the attorneys, and Ms. Armstrong herself. Reconciliation in its very essence is mystery unfolding yet somehow unrevealed. We cannot formulate it or demand it, for reconciliation is intangible and takes many surprising forms. The heart of reconciliation is to begin to heal the very thing that wounded us.

Of course, this is easier said than done. The obstacles that have to be overcome are almost insurmountable. For families that have lost someone to homicide, their world is often shattered and the most familiar things have lost their meaning. Emotions, bills, carry-in dinners, and sympathy cards blur their world. But one thing survivors of homicide often say with acute clarity is: "There is no closure. There is no justice." It is in this dichotomy that I find myself working with families within the judicial system. Regardless of socioeconomic standing, religious beliefs, or education, after a violent loss, families begin a journey with two paths, one of the heart and one of the mind. First, survivors must make sense of their routines and continue with the task of daily living. Second, they experience profound grief and face a hatred that few know. Each person faces this journey differently. The most difficult realization I have made as someone who "walks with," or accompanies, survivors of homicide is that there is no timeline and no road map for their healing. There is a tendency to want to direct the survivor's journey in order to feel helpful. Yet, the most important thing we can do in this role is to validate the grief and questions with acknowledgment but without pre-scribing solutions. By resisting the need to "fix" things, we allow the victim to face these paths honestly. With time, I have seen that the two journeys of heart and mind begin to meet. This meeting is marked with the question, "What do I do with this now?" I can only describe this awareness as a turning.

Roadblocks to Reconciliation

Misunderstanding the Nature of Grieving

> *Every day we struggle to try to remember the beautiful and loving person she was and to drive out the horrible thoughts and visions of how she died. And many times it seemed as though the darkness was stronger than we were, that this terrible deed was so burned into our lives that we would never be able to celebrate who Patricia was. . . . I remember looking at the table we had set out with pho-tographs of her. One that caught my eye was a picture of her at about nine years old looking back over her shoulder with such a sweet expression on her face, and I smiled for the first time remem-bering her as a child.[4]*

—father of a murdered child

Grieving for a loved one who was murdered is not a linear process; rather, it forces a person into a spiral in which the feelings always seem to return around each curve. There are distinctive stages of the mourn-ing process, but public understanding has created the idea that the be-reaved move from A to B to C and so on within set timelines. But experiencing traumatic loss dispels that preconceived notion. Victims who have lost someone to homicide grieve both the loss of their loved one's life and *how* that person died. The sudden and violent nature of death exacerbates emotions or can blunt them for a period of time. The extremity of these emotional and physiological responses can create further instability in a victim's life.

As victims confront their pain, it is often riddled with a blurring of the memory of their loved one. Because the nature of the death was a crime, the emphasis is on the details of their death, not on their life. Surviving family members struggle with anguish, anger, shame, and guilt, which can act as powerful beautifiers. Conversations that should have happened, love that cannot fully bloom, and potential not fully met deprive family members of both remembering the past and honoring the future that their loved one might have had. They counter the horror and loss of control by sanctifying their loved one. I have learned not to judge this process, but to respect it. This tendency is not to deny the humanness of the deceased; it is a demand to recognize it. It is a part of the victim-survivor's healing—bridging the past, their only link to the victim, and integrating the memories into meaning in the survivor's future.

The Glib Call for Reconciliation

Are you ready to forgive him [the murderer]?

—pastor of victim's family

Victims can experience their religious community as a group that places high expectations upon the bereaved. One challenge is the speed with which people expect victims to move through the mourning process. One mother's pastor astounded her when he asked about her readiness to forgive the murderer only three weeks after her daughter's death. The mother, still numb with disbelief of her daughter's death, stopped attending church because of the overture made by the pastor. The expectation of reconciliation is promoted as a morally righteous act that adds to a survivor's sense of shame when she is feeling spiritually depleted. Reconciliation is a word that joins the category of lost meaning. The concept of reconciliation is often difficult to grasp either because the common perception of it is "to restore to harmony"[5] or because of its religious implications. One cannot simply restore harmony after such a senseless loss. People who once used their faith as a foundation find they doubt their faith. Victim-survivors often struggle with the question, "Where was God in all of this?"

It is a healthy tendency to question one's faith in life. Through grappling with our questions, we come to a deeper understanding in our beliefs. It is especially normal to do this when traumatic events shatter our world. Judith Herman, a psychiatrist who works with victims of trauma, teaches that traumatic events destroy the victim's fundamental assumptions about the meaningful order of creation.[6] Survivors need to be allowed the time and space for their doubts regarding faith. What they need most are consistent, steadfast individuals who are willing to listen to painful and unanswerable questions. Instead, what they often end up receiving are glib answers about their loved one being in a better place, or questions that deflect the reality of the trauma and place enormous pressure on the survivor. The push for forgiveness has more to do with our need to tidily wrap up the pain and confusion a murder has caused rather than the genuine concern for the survivor's relationship with God. By testing a person's readiness to forgive the offender, we are burdening their beliefs, not emboldening their faith.

The Unintended Harms of the Judicial System

It was turning into a freak show. Everything was about Benvenuto [offender]. Zach deserved more dignity than that.[7]

—Sy Snarr, mother of a murdered son, Zach

With the judicial system forcing the pain of the victim's death onto the family, and the church distilling the pain with language of forgiveness and reconciliation, it is no wonder the victims receive confusing messages. The courts are based on rules and order. But anyone who has ever experienced the tragic loss of a loved one can tell you that grieving is neither of these—it is messy and defies order. During the trial, judges routinely make it clear that there will be no show of emotion, no outbursts in court, and that anyone in violation of this will be removed from the court. The reason for this is to not prejudice the jury with any show of emotion. But taken to such lengths, it is counterproductive to what has the most potential for reconciliation—for victims and the jury want to see signs of remorse or acknowledgment from the defendant. They want to feel vindicated, and an important step toward this is recognition of their pain by the defendant.

The court knows that there is little, if any, expectation that the defendant will do this at trial. One reason that acknowledgment is not encouraged is because the emphasis of the trial is to argue a person's innocence or guilt. This responsibility falls to the attorneys representing the defendant, and to the government, who represents itself as the victim. The judicial system is not seen as a vehicle for reconciliation—it is a vehicle for retribution. The accused must be held accountable for their actions, and society has the right to safeguard itself from violent offenders. It is important to be prudent with the law and to protect both the victims and the defendant.

But the protection designed by the system denies the very thing that moves individuals closer to reconciliation, either with others, with God, or within themselves. The real victims—the family members—often hope that the trial will bring greater understanding to the circumstances of the crime. The families are disappointed when there is no acceptance of responsibility from the defendant. The victim's family has a need to know the intimate details of the crime. Why did you choose my son? What were my father's last words? How long was she alive? Why didn't you call the police or me if there was a problem? Did he say a prayer before you killed him? Knowing that the horrific circumstances cannot change, it is still the human inclination to understand, to know what happened. For families, knowing the details helps to limit the constant replay of their loved one's death with endless variations that can occur when there is no acknowledgment from the offender. Communities want to feel whole; victims want to be recognized; and most offenders, on some personal level and with work from caring professionals, want to accept responsibility for their actions. This desire to understand and to be understood calls for a more engaged response than the judicial system currently allows.

Under the current approach to murder and death penalty cases, there is a sterile atmosphere in regard to the deceased. Facts are coldly stated, questions arise about the victim's culpability, and the attention is on the accused. Understandably, family members become enraged because their grief is sidestepped in the rush to ensure justice for the accused and for society. Victims wonder, "What about our loss?" The Snarr family, whose son Zachary was killed, believes in the death penalty, but opted for a plea agreement so that the family would not have to face a trial and the years of appeals. Sy Snarr's explanation for her family's decision to go with a plea agreement was due to the judicial emphasis on the offender, rather than on the person who has been killed.

Another example of how the judicial system defies sensitivity to families is when court dates are set, especially for the trial. Families' needs are usually not considered in this process, and many have had to reschedule weddings, family reunions, and workloads in order to be present at the trial. If trial dates have been postponed, victims are often not informed, and appear at court with no explanation of the delay. If families desire to be present at the trial—and most do—they essentially have to put their life on hold until the trial is completed. It is not within the legal system's framework to think about the victims' needs and concerns. This is not to argue that prosecutors or defense attorneys do not care about the outcome or impact on the families, but rather that it is not their purpose to address these issues.

The Expectations of Society

> *We who had lost our daughters found that we were not only re-*
> *sponsible for our own grief, but for the grief of the community.*
> *That's just not fair, but it's the truth. We were responsible for ev-*
> *eryone else feeling okay about this.*[8]

> —mother of two murdered daughters

As the victim begins the sojourn on the two paths, it is crucial to feel safe, to be allowed to remember and mourn, and then to reconnect with others.[9] There is, however, a nuanced societal expectation placed upon survivors to contain their grief, so that somehow their mourning can be done out of view so as to not disrupt the societal flow of work and daily busy-ness. Survivors are expected to rise above their suffering for the common good. As for the legal case against the accused, victims are to show up in court with their dignity intact and defiant of the pain that has been inflicted. Religious institutions want survivors to put their faith in God to carry the burden of their pain; victims may be told that they "cannot fully heal without the power of Christ in their life."[10] Colleagues, friends, and family avoid bereaved ones if they do not follow the American societal pattern for grieving. The expectation is that the mourning is a succinct task with linear confines.[11]

People who have close relationships to victims feel at a loss for what to say or do when a loved one is murdered. Telling someone that we are sorry for their loss seems appropriate the first couple of times we are together. After a while, no longer knowing what to say, we distance ourselves, eventually avoiding contact with the victim. Some friends of victims lose contact permanently, as though the stain of the murder was somehow a falling-out between the victim and themselves. Others try after a time to have a normal relationship with the victims, but they may resume communication as if the lapse in time and the homicide had not happened. Because we are such a "can-do" society and we cannot *undo* what happened to the deceased, we transfer this expectation onto the victim-survivors. This unwillingness to acknowl-edge their loss and to allow victims to fully mourn adds undue burden on the survivors and can stymie their ability to truly make meaning of the forced circumstances of the homicide as well as their ability to reconnect with us.

The Impact of the Media

Moose said sarcastically: "I have not received any message that the citizens of Montgomery County want Channel 9 or The Washington Post or other media outlets to solve this case. . . . If they do, let me know. We will go and do other police work, and we will turn this case over to the media. And you can solve it."[12]

—Chief of Police Charles Moose, regarding the cases
against John Muhammad and Lee Malvo,
accused D.C. area snipers

We have an innate need to understand and to know why crimes happened and what propelled the killers to act as they did. The proof of this is in the paradox of the media's frenzy to report certain crimes and our fascination with the details of them. We want to be invisible witnesses in the search for the killers, investigators during the pre-trial frenzy around the accused, and the jury at trial. We want to hear the confession and the accused's justification for the crime. The community seeks responsibility and remorse from the defendant, like the victim's family does. This is a normal response when harm has been caused within the community. But unlike the victim's family, we experience the tragedy on a superficial level because we are unwilling to confront the pain and because it does not impact our lives long term. We deny that this could happen to us by "othering"; we compare our lives to that of the deceased and try to make distinctions between the two in order to distance ourselves from the possibility of such crimes happening to us. We refuse to accept another person's terror as our own, and we hold the deceased responsible. We ache for the victims' loss, but we minimize it because we do not acknowledge that their loss, in some way, is also our own.

Overcoming the Roadblocks to Reconciliation

Societal Repentance

Repentance is the ability, through God's grace, to start over. It's a new day. We can begin again.[13]

Each day we have the opportunity to start over, to make anew. Earl Zimmerman, a Mennonite pastor said, "We should not be prisoners of our past. We don't need to be tied to our fears, our hatreds, and our regrets."[14] There is enough skill and wisdom from the various professional and lay communities to transform the way survivors are treated after a loved one has been murdered. Our development, both as individuals and as part of a community, depends upon our reaching past set patterns and exploring life beyond our fears and regrets. We have resisted challenges that are unknown to us, and this has limited our growth. By owning our mistakes, repenting, we are given an opportunity for reconciliation with people we have systematically denied.

As a society, we would do well if we took the time to listen to victims as a part of their healing. Trauma creates a need to tell the story again and again. It is telling their truth that provides a catharsis for victims. And it is in listening to this truth that others can be witnesses to their pain. James Gilligan, a psychiatrist who has worked for decades with victims and offenders, wrote, "it is in telling stories that we originally acquired our humanness."[15] Telling the story of their loved one, memorializing the life before their death, is one of the steps in creating meaning for the victim. Jack Shea, a storyteller and hospital chaplain, has said that there are a couple of rules for listening to people whose loved ones have died. First, only the survivor can speak. Next, we as the listener must empty our thoughts or agenda and open our hearts to what the survivor has to say. And finally, the listener must remember that every time is the first time.[16] As a professional or layperson, we may have heard other stories of loss, but we must remember, for this person it is the *first* time they have lost this loved one. There cannot be enough said about the power of listening. Truly listening to a person can awaken in them a deeper understanding of their story.[17]

The "shoulds" for mourning need to be transferred from the victims and onto the community and society. We need to act as a collective model of compassion following a situation that showed no compassion. Each bereaved person is the expert on their pain, but others can be lights in a tunnel of darkness. In fact, survivors will tell you, they *need* others to listen to them, to validate their feelings, and to accompany the person on their journey—to "bear witness" as the process unfolds.[18] We are not responsible for a victim's grief work, but our complicity in denying a public place for their mourning and our unwillingness to embrace the messiness of their grief limits their ability to find ways to reconcile what has happened in their life. Only the survivor can do the healing work, but it cannot be done in isolation. Isolation insulates the bereaved from the very people to whom they need to connect—their community. And when the community creates a space for the victim, it is amazing to witness the grief work in process. It shows me the resilience of the human spirit despite the failings of humanity.

Support people need to embrace the pain without regret. For too long we have separated ourselves from painful situations and people in sorrow. We have created false boundaries to people's pain because we believe our differences will spare us the grief that has come to others. By reestablishing our role in the community, we are nurturing within ourselves the very essence of what it means to be human—to do soul work, to connect with others, and to deepen the meaning of our existence.

Fulfilling Obligations

In the United States, crime is seen as rules that have been broken, rather than harm that has been caused. Howard Zehr, a man who has committed his life work to rethinking crime and its effects, argues that crimes create obligations.[19] Dr. Zehr's work has helped create the philosophy of restorative justice, which reframes the thinking about criminal offenses. Rather than asking the questions, "Who broke the law?" and "What do they deserve?" restorative justice asks the questions, "Who has been hurt?" "What are their needs?" and "Whose responsibility is it to meet these needs?" Asking the questions differently creates an expansive approach that shifts the focus from only the defendant to also include the victim and the community. Restorative justice broadens the emphasis from only retribution for the defendant to include the needs and obligations of *all* parties affected by the crime.

With a restorative justice approach, obligations are hemmed into the very fabric of the criminal case because of the harm that has been caused to the victim, the family, and the community. Obligations start with embracing the surviving family members, hearing their needs, and addressing their concerns. It is from this foundation that all other actions should emerge. Regardless of whether the offender and the victim knew one another, the crime forced a relationship onto the parties. As mentioned earlier, victims have questions about the crime and concerns about the outcome that only the defendant can answer. More than any other role within the judicial system, the relationship between the victim and the offender has an organic bond that cannot be changed by the government acting as the victim or by the defense throwing doubt on the culpability of their client. The law provides protections from that relationship, but it also restricts it. Healing takes place when the legal system provides the opportunity for the defendant to accept responsibility and when both parties' needs are addressed. It is the road back to humanity.

The Judicial System

The day after Sheila Rockwell met for three hours with her son's killer, Chris Dean, she took the stand to give her victim impact statement at Mr. Dean's sentencing hearing. She talked of the loss she felt with her son's death; her inability to walk without crutches or to write because of the physical injuries she sustained in the bomb's explosion; she talked of the good things her son did like train dogs for the blind and rescue greyhounds from extermination. She gave life to the memory of her son who had now been dead for a year and a half. As she stood to leave the stand, Chris Dean looked at Ms. Rockwell and said in an audible tone, "I am so sorry." Sheila Rockwell walked back to her seat in the gallery and as she moved past Chris Dean's wife, Diane, Diane held her hand out to Sheila. The two women held hands for several minutes until the judge called for a recess so that the courtroom could regain its composure.[20]

The judicial system is an excellent place to bridge compassion with justice. Despite the legal system's attempt to extract emotion and base its judgment on law, the courts are a place that can be the start of redemption. The concern for protecting the rights of the accused and upholding the law does not have to come at the loss of such powerful possibilities for those impacted by the crime. Although the legal system works on the assumption that it needs to shield the victims from the defendant, on an organic level, it is this very relationship that holds this promise.

Through formal channels within the judicial system, the victims can express their questions, concerns, and judicial needs. Using the same means, the defendant can address the victims' needs and personal concerns for the future. Attorneys can use their negotiation skills to navigate this process, but they would need to reorient their idea of success. To do this, attorneys need to move away from a distributive bargaining position and take a more integrative negotiation approach.[21] Prosecutors use the law to seek justice; defense attorneys use it to seek mercy, but neither of these should be mutually exclusive. The tendency within the legal community has been that in order to come out first, only one's own interests can triumph in the courtroom. Integrative negotiation offers an opportunity to secure interests for all parties that impact their lives beyond the trial.

Unfortunately, it is not always possible to negotiate every legal case. That being said, attorneys are still in the greatest position to be models of compassion during the judicial proceedings. Balancing professionalism, zealous advocacy, and respect for the memory of the deceased as well as for the family members makes for good lawyering no matter what side the attorney represents. I have seen the profound impact an attorney's actions can have on the family as well as the rest of the courtroom when they incorporate awareness of how trials affect people's lives, and their effort is worthwhile. The legal system is necessary in order to maintain safety and as a structure for accountability, but again, neither of these need to exist in a vacuum void of humanity. Rather, it is when the courts allow a space for acknowledgment that invested individuals begin to reconnect with society, their community, and their lives.

Witness to Resurrection

This forgiveness does not seem to be something I have won or earned . . . it is a gift of grace.[22]

—father of murdered daughter

Reconciliation begins in a mysterious way—it is hard to know whether it starts in one's own heart or with one's God. For families who have lost a loved one to homicide, it is almost a resurrection more than reconciliation, with a seamless line between the two. In the months and years that follow the homicide, victims do not believe that there will be a day that their heart will not ache. It seems inconceivable that they would go a day without crying or thinking about their child, sister, or husband. But time, grieving, and mystery often defy the enormity of their loss. As mentioned earlier, there often comes a point in a survivor's life in which something turns. Sometimes the turning is so gradual that one has to deliberately trace back one's pain to see how far they have come in their healing. And sometimes, the shift is profound and memorable. Bud Welch recalled the first time he saw Bill McVeigh, the father of Timothy McVeigh, on the news. Something began to shift in how he felt about losing his daughter in the Oklahoma City bombing.

When I saw him on television, I recognized that man's pain. He is
hurting as much as I am. The reporters didn't give him the same
privacy as they gave the survivors of the bombing. They treated
him like he deserved the intrusion. But it was when I saw his pain,
I realized he has lost a son, like I lost a daughter.[23]

This change created a need in Bud to meet Bill. He needed to connect
with the humanity he saw in another parent. A couple of years after the
bombing, Bud was in New York and went about seeing if he could meet
Bill McVeigh. Bill agreed and directions to his house were given to Bud.
When Bud arrived at the house, the two men stood in the driveway awk-
wardly searching their minds for what to say. "Want to see my garden?"
Bill asked. The two men spent hours talking about farming, raising children, and very little about the bombing. On his way back to the hotel, Bud
called me. This is what I remember from our conversation: Bill was proud
of his strawberries; Bud was crying so hard I worried about his ability to
drive the car, and he said, "Tammy, he is a working Joe just like I am."[24]

A victim-survivor's resurrection is often slow and tedious. Homicide
takes away everything you took for granted. Lynn Shiner, a mother whose
two children were killed by her ex-husband, explains it like this:

I can't reorder anything, because if I did, I would just pick up the
scrambled pieces and put them back in order. It's more like all the
rungs on a ladder are removed. I'm at the bottom and have to start
all over. You build, you create a new life. I have a couple of pieces
from my old life that I have to fit in.[25]

Rebuilding a life after a tragic event is an integrated process of the
journey of the heart and mind. Victims rebuild their lives out of necessity,
not as a triumph over adversity. They long to have their lives as they were
before their loved one was murdered, and would do anything to change
the circumstances. But life poses the challenge, "How do you want to
live?" and it is from here that victims begin to walk the turning path.

When a person agrees to accompany someone on their journey of healing, they make the commitment to let go of the perceived idea of time for
grieving and healing. In order to "bear witness"[26] to a person's journey,
one embraces the reality of accompanying that person for a long time.
Many may have assumed that Leslie Armstrong, whose story opened this
chapter, transcended her pain over the death of her daughter Joie at Cary
Stayner's sentencing hearing. But it would be disingenuous of me to sug-

gest that. After the judicial proceedings, Leslie struggled with severe depression, anxiety, and shame. She experienced feelings of rage and loss that no one should have to know. It was difficult to watch her. It was harder to hear her pain and know that there was nothing I could do to "fix" it. There were times when Leslie could not have contact with me because our connection started with the tragic end of Joie's life and this association brought too many strong feelings. But my commitment was to Leslie and to accompany her regardless of the difficult times.

Until I met Leslie, I believed reconciliation could happen but that no one could determine how or when. As I watched Leslie plummet into the dark abyss of memories, clothing, jewelry, and questions, I began to think that I did not understand enough about tragedy and how it could break the human spirit. In September 2002, Leslie and I were talking on a Sunday evening, after not having had contact for several months. She was telling me of the horse farm that she and her friend Hammie had just purchased. Leslie was jubilant as she talked of her plans to board horses and to work with local youth clubs at her farm. She had begun tutoring students in math in a neighborhood that desperately needed the loving attention of a person like her. At one point she said, "You know that I would give it all up and go back to my crummy job if I could have Joie back." "You know that you don't even need to say that," is all that I could muster.[27] As she talked, tears streamed down my cheeks because I was given the gift of witnessing Leslie's death and resurrection. Reconciliation. Whatever you want to call it.

The possibilities for reconciliation come in many forms. It can take place with oneself, with one's God, and even with the offender. Not all stories end like the ones I have shared, but I offer them to show that the possibilities are real. It is my hope that the people who have lost someone to homicide, and their stories, can act as a guiding point for change within our society and judicial system. For when reconciliation happens, it is not something you expect, rather something you hope against hope for in your heart. And when you witness it, you are in the presence of grace. It is a holy place to be.

Notes

1. This quote is compiled from the following three sources: Associated Press, "Yosemite Killer Ducks Death Penalty with Plea Bargain," *Daily News-Record* (1 December 2000); Jerry Bier and Matthew Kreamer, "Stayner Gets Life, Killer Cries as He Apologizes to the Armstrong Family," *The Fresno Bee* (1 December 2000); Christine Hanley, "At His Sentencing, Yosemite Killer Apologizes to Family," *Los Angeles Times* (1 December 2000).

2. Ibid.

3. I want to thank the families that I have worked with, whose stories give meaning to this chapter. Leslie Armstrong, Sheila Rockwell, and Bud Welch allowed me the grace to walk with them on their journeys and to share their stories here.

4. Hector Black, transcript of *State of Georgia v. Ivan Christopher Simpson* (Georgia Superior Court: 14 January 2002), 25–26.

5. *Merriam Webster's Collegiate Dictionary*, Tenth Edition (Springfield, MA: Merriam Webster, 1996).

6. Judith Lewis Herman, *Trauma and Recovery* (New York: Basic Books, 1992), 51.

7. Stephen Hunt, "Death Penalty Often Dropped in Exchange for Peace of Mind," *Salt Lake City Tribune* (30 September 2002).

8. Howard Zehr, *Transcending: Reflections of Crime Victims* (Intercourse, PA: Good Books, 2001), 20.

9. Herman, *Trauma and Recovery*.

10. "Foundation for Healing: A Personal Relationship with Jesus Christ," 1999, GriefShare, Church Initiative, 2 January 2003, at www.griefrecovery.com/pages/foundation.html.

11. There is a common misperception of Elizabeth Kübler-Ross's original work on the stages of grieving. Some hold the perspective that these stages are distinct *and* linear, but many caregivers know that was not the intention of Kübler-Ross's work. One person who has written about this topic is Dr. Alan Wolfelt; see www.centerforloss.com.

12. Josh White, Jamie Stockwell, and Michael Ruane, "Prince William Police Probe Sniper Link in Shooting" *Washington Post* (10 October 2002).

13. Earl Zimmerman, sermon, "The Beginning of the Beginning" (Harrisonburg, VA: Shalom Mennonite Church, 8 December 2002).

14. Ibid.

15. James Gilligan, *Violence: Reflections on a National Epidemic* (New York: Vintage, 1997), 4.

16. John Shea, speech, Associated Brethren Caregivers (Elizabethtown, PA: Elizabethtown College, June 1999).

17. For more information about this topic, read Elise Boulding, *Building a Global Civic Culture: Education for an Interdependent World* (Syracuse, NY: Syracuse University Press, 1990).

18. Sandra Bloom, *Creating Sanctuary* (New York: Routledge, 1997), 246–47.

19. For more information about restorative justice, read Howard Zehr's books: *Changing Lenses* (Scottdale, PA: Herald Press, 1990), and *The Little Book of Restorative Justice* (Intercourse, PA: Good Books, 2002).

20. Sheila Rockwell, telephone conversations, February 2000, January 2003.

21. R.J. Lewicki, D.A. Saunders, and J. Minton, *Essentials of Negotiation*, 2d ed. (Burr Ridge, IL: Irwin McGraw Hill, 2000).

22. Leon Alligood. "Jackson County Quaker asks court to spare killed of woman he helped raise," *The Tennessean* (26 December 2002).

23. Bud Welch, telephone conversation, May 1997.

24. Bud Welch, telephone conversation, June 1999.

25. Zehr, *Transcending: Reflections of Crime Victims*, 9.

26. Ibid.

27. Leslie Armstrong, telephone conversation, September 2002.

September 11

Clash of Civilizations or Islamic Revolution?

Richard C. Martin

Recently, "Morning Edition" of National Public Radio (NPR) stopped people in the Washington, D.C., suburbs on their way to work or school and asked them about their perception of Islam and violence. One woman caught my attention when she told the reporter that it was not Islam as such, but the Wahhabis whose violence and extremism were threatening world order. This was a variation on the "good Muslims versus bad Muslims" dichotomy that we have heard so much about from our national leaders and the media: most Muslims are good; Osama bin Laden and Wahhabis are bad. But that was not what caught my attention most. The woman's remark struck me as a refinement on the widely discussed "Clash of Civilizations" thesis advanced by Harvard political scientist Samuel P. Huntington a decade ago. Her interpretation was unusual in the fact that it came not from a pundit or a specialist in Islamic studies. It came from a middle-class citizen who probably has cable television and access to the Web. It indicates that since September 11 we as a society have had almost unlimited access to information about Islam— much more so than we did following the Iranian Revolution and the taking of American hostages in 1979, or the Gulf War in 1991. This may be a consequence of more than a year of 24–7 cable news focus (and a plethora of new websites) on Islam. Dispensing knowledge about Islam and terrorism has become a gigantic growth industry in this country, including in our universities, and a lot of entrepreneurs have risen to serve this lucrative industry and profit from it. Lost in much of this glut of portrayals of Islam is that there are serious disputes among Muslim intellectuals and activists about what Islam means in the world we live in. Some of the issues are as difficult and deeply conflicted, say, as the pro-choice/pro-life debate among Christians and others.

The purpose of this chapter is to join the conversation in this volume about the role of religion in reconciliation, or the possibility of reconciliation in religiously inspired conflicts, with particular reference to competing religious interpretations and social movements among Muslims. The argument steers us away from analyzing world events involving Islam in terms of the good Muslim/bad Muslim dichotomy, despite the obvious fact that a good many Muslims and not a few non-Muslims have tried to nail Osama bin Laden, al-Qaeda, and Wahhabis as bad Muslims. The discussion that follows will mention but not pursue the urgent need for reconciliation between Muslims and non-Muslims in such instances as the violent flare-ups between local Muslim and Christian communities in Nigeria, Egypt, Pakistan, and Indonesia. The main argument of this chapter is that the events of September 11 and their aftermath have exposed sharply conflicting theological interpretations and sociopolitical identities among Muslims in the world today, and in many cases these conflicts have deep historical roots. The focus is on the need for reconciliation among Muslims themselves, between modern globalized Wahhabi or Salafi movements among Sunni Muslims and more local and historically rooted communities of Sunni and Shi'ite Muslims in Asia, Africa, Europe, and the Americas. A secondary area of need for reconciliation is among Muslim and non-Muslim Americans, especially following two years of legal and illegal harassment of Muslims or anyone who looks Muslim either under the cover of the Patriot Act and the Department of Homeland Security or, in most cases, out of simple ignorance and fear of the other. In both cases, reconciliation will not come easily or quickly. It will require learning about what for most Americans is the Other, Islam. Our point of departure is the recognition that in order to work toward reconciliation we must first understand the issues in conflict and the theological expressions of those issues.

Furthermore, it is necessary to understand the dispute among scholars in the academy over the past two decades about how to explain and interpret Islamist groups and especially the more activist and strident reform movements. In a collection of published articles titled *Islam, Politics and Social Movements*, based on a conference in 1981 just following the Iranian Revolution, the editors, Ira Lapidus and Edmund Burke III, asked contributors to explore the problematic of whether Islamic fundamentalism should be understood as Islamic politics or as a social movement. According to Lapidus, neo-orientalists (Islam specialists) argue that the task of understanding Islamist activities in the Muslim world is to analyze Islamic rhetoric, symbols, and interpretations used by insurgent movements "in different political and economic settings throughout the Muslim world." In other words, in order to understand Islamic social movements, the focus must be on Islam as such. Those social scientists who reject the neo-orientalist approach are more concerned to show "how social protest arises and especially . . . the social and political structures within which such movements arise, regardless of the cultural idiom in which such grievances are expressed."[1] Burke put it more succinctly: "Is it *Islamic* political movements? Or *social* movements in Islamic societies?"[2] Burke and Lapidus, and many of the scholars contributing to their volume, make the point that the question as posed is unproductive. The two approaches must be reconciled if we are to develop effective and accurate understandings of what the woman interviewed by NPR identified, accurately I think, as a potential problem in the Muslim world, namely Wahhabism. I will not go into the dispute between neo-orientalists and social movement theorists further, except to point out that much of the writing and TV commentary about Islam since September 11 seems to operate on one or the other side of this debate. A methodology that combines both kinds of analyses is what some scholars have tried to develop during the past decade.[3]

Most interesting is the popular view among many Muslim and Western scholars—and now also among ordinary consumers of media—that Wahhabism as such is dangerous, un-Islamic, and an aberration from acceptable variations of Sunni Islam. I want to applaud that NPR interviewee for grasping the fact that the term Wahhabi has an important reference in Islam. At the same time, I will try to complicate and frustrate the tendency in public discourse to construct simplistic distinctions between "good Islam" and "bad Islam." Whether or not it will be possible for Muslim intellectuals to achieve a reconciliation of Wahhabism or the so-called Wahhabi movement in Islam with more traditional, as well as liberal, progressive, and even Shi'ite interpretations cannot be answered here.

Clash of Civilizations

Let me begin with the Huntington thesis of a Clash of Civilizations and then put that in perspective before moving to another approach I think we must take. A growing number of historians and political scientists have seen in September 11 a confirmation that Islam is a violence-prone religion that is on a collision course with Western civilization and with the United States in particular. Among the most distinguished members of that school of interpretation are the historian Bernard Lewis, the political scientist Samuel P. Huntington, the social theorist Francis Fukuyama, and the writer V.S. Naipaul. This is the "Islam is a world problem" school of thought, and its views are now prevalent in the media, in journal and book scholarship, and indeed in the classroom. Of growing concern to many scholars is the fact that this view in the academy has encouraged an air of vigilantism to hunt down and expose faculty and others who write and teach about Islam in constructive ways. The American Council of Trustees and Alumni, founded in December 2001 by Lynne Cheney, the former head of the National Endowment for the Humanities and wife of Vice President Richard Cheney, and by Senator Joseph Lieberman, published a document in which they identified in the late fall of 2001 some 117 examples of anti-American faculty whose writings and classroom lectures present critiques of U.S. foreign policy and constructive statements about Islamic culture and Muslims—which Cheney and Lieberman interpreted as anti-American in light of September 11.

More recently, Daniel Pipes, with moral support from Cheney and scholars such as Bernard Lewis, Martin Kramer, the *National Review*, and other right-wing organs of opinion, has ratcheted up the vigilantism process by publishing new lists with specific charges against specific faculty in Islamic studies. Their website (www.campus-watch.org) has encouraged "patriotic" students to report to Campus Watch any professor or course that is critical of U.S. foreign policy in the Muslim world or that attempts to explain why many Muslims, abroad and at home, express anger toward America. The result has been rather chilling for those of us who have come to see our task as teaching the skills of critical thinking. Even more recently, Jerry Falwell has revitalized the ancient Byzantine polemical genre of attacking the character and morals of the Prophet Muhammad. In this he is followed by other Islamophobic Protestant evangelists, such Pat Robertson, host of the popular TV show "700 Club," and Franklin Graham, son of the Rev. Billy Graham. These are religious leaders who are listened to and respected by perhaps hundreds of thousands of followers. That they insist on retailing false information about Islam and Muslims, devoid of any scholarly truth or integrity, has the effect of frustrating dialogue and understanding among American Muslims and Christians.

Other scholars and writers have argued variations of a countertheory and explanation about Islam in world history, namely, that it is a vastly and perhaps deliberately misunderstood civilization, demonized and misrepresented in Western scholarship, which fails to recognize the potential in Islam to provide some of the solutions to the world's problems. Among the best known writers in this camp are scholars such as Bruce Lawrence, author of *Shattering the Myth: Islam Beyond Violence*,[4] and John Esposito, author of *The Islamic Threat: Myth or Reality?*[5] These are the defenders of Islam, the mostly non-Muslim scholars, often with Christian or Jewish identities, who, in the climate of the times, have sought to challenge what they see as false and misleading representations of Islam and have put themselves in the service of its rescue.

Like the defenders of Islam, I think it is necessary to challenge the "Islam is a world problem" school. Following Boston University anthropologist Robert Hefner, I would like to suggest that what we may be seeing in the Middle East, Africa, South Asia, and elsewhere in the Islamic world is a reformation (one might even argue a revolution), a postcolonial struggle for power and Islamic identity in the face of multinational globalization and tectonic shifts in military, economic, and cultural power happening in the world today.[6] In making this argument, I avoid the role of trying to defend Islam. It is not my purpose to construct a reactive scholarship that answers Islam's cultured (and uncultured) despisers. Moreover, Islam does not need me to defend it. It has intellectuals and scholars serious of purpose who can do so much better and more authentically. To understand better the "bad Islam" side of the equation, we need to return to the critics of Islam, but this time to more serious scholars and public intellectuals, or the "Islam is a world problem" group.[7]

The "Islam Is a World Historical Problem" Argument

It is easy to dismiss the vituperative remarks made about Islam by V.S. Naipaul on February 22, 2002, at a literary conference in India, in which he managed to insult Hindus, Muslims, feminists, postcolonial theorists, and practically everyone else.[8] His Hindu colleagues called him rude and found it impossible to try to have a conversation with him during the conference. His longstanding criticism of Islam was published, *inter alia*, in two books: *Among the Believers* (1981) and *Beyond Belief* (1998).[9] These have been widely read in the English-speaking world and have drawn a great deal of critical acclaim as well as not a small amount of negative criticism. I had the distinction of traveling to three of the four countries Naipaul wrote about in *Among the Believers* a couple of years after he published his book and of meeting many of the same people he had interviewed in Pakistan, Malaysia, and Indonesia. (In case you might be wondering, my own impressions of the people he met and wrote about were very different from his.)

Naipaul's earlier thesis that Islam, especially fundamentalist Islam, has been a constant source of religious and communal violence in the contemporary world has found some other notable supporters. Another troubling intellectual contribution to the critique of Islam came in 1989, this time from an academic, with the publication by Francis Fukuyama of an article titled "The End of History and the Last Man," published in the *National Interest*, and later expanded and published as a book of the same title by the Free Press in New York in 1992. Fukuyama argued the Hegelian thesis that universal progress through history would soon leave liberal democracy as the highest order of human society. In this line of argument, Fukuyama understands radical Islamist Muslims as today's new breed of what he unabashedly terms "Islamo-Fascists." Sticking with his Hegelian dialectic, Fukuyama argues that radical, anti-liberal movements in Islam, given to violence and social disorder, will in time soon be overcome by liberal and modernist movements, toward which he believes Islamic history is necessarily evolving.[10]

Among those who wrote approvingly of Fukuyama's earlier work was the Harvard political scientist Samuel P. Huntington. In the summer of 1993, Huntington contributed a now infamous article to the Washington, D.C., journal *Foreign Affairs* titled "The Clash of Civilizations." Close readers of this line of scholarship have pointed out that Huntington derived this arresting title from an article that Princeton historian Bernard Lewis wrote over a decade ago. In "The Roots of Muslim Rage," published in the *Atlantic Monthly*,[11] Lewis concluded that in the aftermath of reactions against Salman Rushdie's *Satanic Verses*, "we are facing a mood and a movement far transcending the level of issues and policies and the governments that pursue them. This is no less than a clash of civilizations—the perhaps irrational but surely historic reaction of an ancient rival against our Judeo-Christian heritage, our secular present, and the worldwide expansion of both." Lewis goes on to warn Western readers, appropriately enough, that "it is crucially important that we on our side should not be provoked into an equally historic but equally irrational reaction against that rival."[12] But that balancing cautionary note has been lost in Lewis's quickly produced post-September 11 book, *What Went Wrong?*[13]

This phenomenon of finding Islamic civilization prone toward violence and therefore ethically deficient in such concepts as just-war theory, is what John Kelsay calls "putting Islam in the dock." A few years ago during the height of the war in Bosnia, Kelsay wrote an essay in which he chided Bernard Lewis and other critics who are taken seriously in Washington and in the national media. According to Kelsay, in writing about Islam in order to influence American foreign policy, Lewis and others "are no longer dealing strictly in matters of policy; they are making normative judgments about Islamic tradition."[14]

Along with such American colleagues as John Esposito, Bruce Lawrence, and John Kelsay, I believe that Western intellectuals have something to learn from Islamic history and Muslim intellectuals about ethics and society. The tired criticisms of Islamic civilization as inherently (or more recently) violent and driven to dominate the rest of the world go back very far in history; Naipaul, Huntington, and Lewis are just the most recent purveyors of this critique. My major criticism of Esposito, Lawrence, and other non-Muslim defenders of Islam in the present debate about a clash of civilizations is that we must not try to defend, or even allow ourselves to be understood as trying to defend, a counter-thesis which claims that Islamic civilization is entirely innocent of violence against the other or of the misuse of power. The game of debate must not be allowed to blind us to the misuses of power and of actions taken, sometimes driven by religious conviction, that have led to great social injustices. Islamic history, like Western and Eastern Christian history, and Asian Confucian history, is replete with examples, such as the Thirty Years War in Europe, that require us as intellectuals and moral beings to condemn all such acts of violence and inhumanity against other humans. Now, however, addressing the problem of terrorism and its causes is a matter of global necessity, not simply a matter of national interest under the control of the National Security advisors to President Bush at the White House.

Islamic Reformation

There is an alternative to the interpretation of the events leading to September 11 and the discoveries of deep-seated anti-Western feelings in the Muslim world as a "clash of civilizations." Several years ago, graffiti and posters began to appear in public spaces in Islamic countries bearing the slogan *al-Islam huwa al-hall*—"Islam is the solution." The problems for which Islam could be seen to be a solution were well known in many parts of the Muslim world. One needed only to visit any bookstore in Cairo or Jakarta to find prominently displayed the writings of twentieth-century Islamists like the Indian-Pakistani ideologue Abu l-A'la al-Mawdudi and the Egyptian Islamist Sayyid Qutb, who was put to death in Cairo by the Egyptian government in 1971, nearly a decade before the Iranian Revolution. Their writings are also available in this country in English. Although they do not yet occupy a very large place in curriculum on Islam in American higher education, they are being read in curricula at some universities that offer courses beyond the introductory survey course on Islam.

Mawdudi was the founder of the Islamic reform and proselytism movement known as the Jam'at-i Islami that has become popular among South Asian and other Muslim students.[15] The problems he saw in South Asia in the mid-twentieth century were the moral and social failures of the great Western ideologies in the twentieth century: communism, socialism, and capitalism. These failures were grounded in the spiritual bankruptcy of European and American society, about which the Egyptian Sayyid Qutb wrote eloquently in his famous revolutionary little book, *Ma'alim fi al-tariq* (Milestones Along the Way).[16] The milestones Qutb wanted Muslims to see were the signs of the failure of post-Enlightenment secularism, such as racism in America (which Sayyid Qutb experienced firsthand), the sexual revolution (which also embarrassed and offended him during his visit to America in the early 1950s), and the dwindling spiritual authority of religion in public life. For Mawdudi, Qutb, the Muslim Brotherhood, and other Islamic revival movements, the only solution for modern humankind was Islam, a return to the teachings and practices of Islam as introduced by the Prophet Muhammad and established in the first three generations, known as the Salaf. The modern Arabic term *salafi* refers to those Muslims whose faith and practice is modeled on the Salaf. Salafi Islam is a global movement, thanks primarily to information technology.[17] Those Muslims who are critical of the sharp boundaries Salafi Muslims draw around Islamic faith and practice and their methods of spreading their interpretation of Islam often refer to them as "Wahhabis." The term Wahhabi has a particular historical reference, as we shall see below, but like the woman interviewed on NPR, it is often used these days by Muslims and non-Muslims alike as a term of opprobrium.

The Salafi tradition within Islam became historically embodied primarily in one of the four Sunni legal schools of interpretation (*madhhab*), known as the Hanbalis, who took their name from the great traditionalist, Ahmad ibn Hanbal (d. 855). In 833, ibn Hanbal, along with a number of other Muslim jurists, was called before the Caliph al-Ma'mun to publicly renounce the popular traditionalist doctrine that the Qur'an, the Muslim scripture, was the eternal and uncreated Word of God. Al-Ma'mun and the court theologians reasoned that the Qur'an was created, like the ink and paper on which it was written and the sound waves and organs of speech and hearing by which it was heard. To say otherwise, these theologians argued, was to postulate the existence of a second eternal being with God, which was particularly unacceptable in Islamic conceptions of monotheism.

Ibn Hanbal, however, was a public figure deeply respected among the masses in Iraq for his piety and his unflinching devotion to the Qur'an as the eternal word of God. He became an icon for the deep reverence Muslims in all generations have felt toward the Arabic Qur'an. His piety and refusal to say the Qur'an was created (leading to his imprisonment with large demonstrations for his release outside) is sometimes compared to Martin Luther's "Here I Stand" speech in response to the Holy See's demand that he recant his criticisms of the Roman Church. Hanbalism (in Arabic *hanabila*) developed after his death into not only a Sunni school of legal interpretation, known as the Hanbali *madhhab* or scholarly trend in interpretation, but also into what some scholars regard as a social movement. In early Islam, a variety of local schools arose in the lands where Islam spread, usually around a respected teachers like ibn Hanbal. By the tenth (fourth Islamic) century, the differences in interpretation among Sunni Muslims had narrowed to four major trends, of which Hanbalism was one. It eventually came to exert the greatest influence in the Arabian Peninsula and the Gulf region. The Shafi'i and Hanafi *madhhab*s competed with each other in the central Islamic lands of West Asia and have continued to maintain a presence there, but the more liberal Hanafi school of interpretation predominated in two great centers of learning in the Middle East, Turkey (Ottoman Empire) and Egypt (al-Azhar University), while the Shafi'i school has predominated in the populous lands of Southeast Asian Islam. The Maliki School predominated in medieval Spain and spread throughout Africa. In addition to these four Sunni schools, the Imami, Isma'ili, and Zaydi Shi'ite Muslims also developed their own authoritative interpretive traditions.

In medieval Islam, especially in Baghdad, the followers of Ahmad ibn Hanbal were often behind those reform movements in Islam that worried about and reacted, sometimes violently, to popular and non-Muslim religious practices.[18] Intercommunal honoring of religious feast days and visits to shrines were among the targets of puritanical reform efforts.[19] We can trace this theological sentiment against any practice not attributable to the Salaf generations of early Islam through the Hanbali line down to the writings of ibn Taymiyya in the fourteenth century, Muhammad ibn 'Abd al-Wahhab in Arabia in the eighteenth century, and the Muslim Brotherhood in Egypt in the twentieth century. The doctrine of the eternal Qur'an remains deeply embedded in Sunni Muslim thought; ironically, it finds its strongest theological articulation in the prevailing Ash'arite school of theology, which otherwise has been in intellectual conflict with Hanbali theologians. However, the spirit of reform and purification of Islamic practice of modern and non-Muslim accretions, which is widespread in the Islamic world today, is often an expression of the Hanbali interpretation of Islam. It should be understood, however, that the spirit of reform has many expressions besides Hanbalism among intellectuals, professionals, journalists, and students.

In the early modern period, the most ambitious and aggressive reform movement has often gone by the label "Wahhabism," named after the aforementioned spiritual founder of Saudi Arabia, Muhammad ibn 'Abd al-Wahhab (1703–1787). He adopted a strong Hanbali belief that Islamic practice in eighteenth-century Arabia deviated from the true religion as taught and practiced by the Prophet Muhammad and the Salaf. A prince of the al-Saud family befriended 'Abd al-Wahhab, and the two leaders forged the beginning of the kingdom that was to become the modern Saudi state in the twentieth century. In the eighteenth century the al-Saud family delivered the Nejd (the region in the east around modern Riyadh) from Ottoman control, and Wahhabi Puritanism purged Islamic practice of popular and syncretic expressions of Islam, including Sufi mystical worship. The Wahhabi movement survived Muhammad ibn 'Abd al-Wahhab's death and became the prevailing religious world view in Arabia and eventually the modern Gulf states, although other Hanbali scholars and reformers were sharply critical, especially of the Wahhabi tendency toward strident verbal and even physical attacks on other Muslims. They worried about the narrow boundaries that Wahhabism put on the Islamic faith, which had the effect of sharply dividing Wahhabi Muslims not only from other religions, but also, and more importantly, from other Muslims. The Hanbali spirit of cleansing Islam of foreign beliefs and practices, then, was revived in the eighteenth century by the Wahhabi reforms, which, it should be noted, were not directed against the West. The colonial power opposed by the Saud family and Muhammad ibn 'Abd al-Wahhab was the Islamic Ottoman Empire, which by the eighteenth century had become a corrupt absentee landlord. Nonetheless, the Wahhabi revival on the eve of European imperialism and colonialism was to inspire reform movements, like the Muslim Brotherhood of Egypt in the twentieth century, that aggressively sought to steer Islam away from Western religious, secular, and political influences.

The Salafiyya as a Social Movement

In the remainder of this chapter I will return to the contemporary usage of the term *salafi*, which is derived from an Arabic root meaning "to precede." Although religious leaders and rulers in Saudi Arabia accept the label "Wahhabi" with pride as followers of the religious teachings of Muhammad ibn 'Abd al-Wahhab, the Salafi movement is now global in scope, operating in most parts of the world where Islam exists, and many Muslims who identify themselves as "Salafi" reject the label "Wahhabi." In its broader usage, Salafi refers to the followers of the Egyptian reformer and modernist Muhammad 'Abduh (d. 1905), who like other reformers taught that a proper understanding of Islam must go back to early Islam and the practice of the Salaf. My use of the term "Salafi" hereafter attempts to avoid the negative connotations the term "Wahhabi" has for some Muslims, even though many researchers use the terms Wahhabi and Salafi interchangeably. More recently than 'Abduh, Salafi Muslims have tended to argue that later generations acquired understandings of Islam that were distorted and sullied by the introduction of innovations (known as *bid'a*), which led to communal fractiousness and falling away from the Sirat al-Mustaqim, the Straight Path of Islam.

Among the things that Salafis have objected to most strenuously are the popular celebration of the birthday of the Prophet Muhammad (because it tends to deify and glorify Muhammad the man over God and the Qur'an); Sufi practices; visiting saints' tombs; and mixing Christian, Hindu, and other religious celebrations with Islamic life. The Salafis have rejected not only the Shi'i and Sufi variations of Islamic interpretation, they have also rejected the notion that there are four *madhhabs*, or acceptable legal schools of interpretation of Islamic law, the Shari'a. A Muslim colleague related to me recently that when she met an Egyptian who expressed very strict and narrow religious beliefs, she asked him what his *madhhab* (school of interpretation) was. He replied that he followed no *madhhab*, but rather that he was a Salafi.[20] For the Salafis there is only one interpretation and one form of practice of Islam, namely, the one they subscribe to. The Salafi movement, or at least some groups affiliated with it, is based on a vision and a hope of creating a transnational community of true believers.

It is important to emphasize that the Salafi approach has clashed with many other Islamic sects and movements. I have mentioned the Sufis. Sufism was the main vehicle for the historical spread of Islam to many parts of Asia and Africa. As Central Asia opened up and began to return to pre-communist religious affiliation, including Islam, Salafi missionaries from the Middle East and South Asia often cause divisions between the imams who follow the older, more mystical practices of Islam that survived the decades of communism in the twentieth century and younger Muslims who seek a strong Islamic identity. The Salafi influence is also very strong, and often divisive, in North America. Thus, the Salafi movement does not seek ecumenical rapprochement with the larger Islamic world. Believing as they do that there is only one accurate religious truth as revealed in the Qur'an and exemplified in practice by the Prophet Muhammad, and that they alone are true to the teachings and practices of Muhammad and his Companions, many Salafis claim that they are the only Muslims who will be saved on Judgment Day. The purpose of jihad for the Salafis is to spread the true belief to the rest of the Muslim world. Rhetorically, the West and modernity are also the targets of the Salafi message, which the Western media have picked up on. It is more important to notice, however, that like Wahhabism in the eighteenth century, the Salafi interpretation primarily targets Islam. It is led by a loose confederation of lay intellectuals and activists who call themselves the vanguard and seek no less than to reform and remake the rest of the Islamic world.

The Salafiyya and Jihad

These religious identity markers are easy to locate in the recent speeches and writings of Osama bin Laden and the movement that has been called al-Qaeda (from *al-qa'ida*, the base, foundation). Within the Salafi movement, bin Laden and his followers represent what has been referred to as the jihadi Salafis—those who advocate the use of force against enemy threats to Islam, such as the Soviet invasion of Afghanistan, the Serbian atrocities against Muslims in the Balkans, the American forces in Somalia, and the continuing presence of U.S. and other Western military forces in Saudi Arabia, contaminating the holy cities of Mecca and Medina. In the latter part of the twentieth century, several groups arose, such as Islamic Jihad and Hezbollah, which did advocate violent forms of jihad for specific causes. By and large, however, the Islamist reform movements inspired by the writings of ibn Taymiyya, Mawdudi, and Sayyid Qutb did not preach the use of violence in the spread of Islam and encounters with the non-Muslim world.

Majid Khaddouri, John Kelsay, and other scholars have shown that the classical jurists in Islam paid considerable attention to what just war theorists refer to as *jus in bello* (legitimate means of violence in war), but much less attention to *jus ad bellum* (the grounds for going to war). Indeed, in the beginning stages of the Soviet war in Afghanistan, the call for Muslims to go to Afghanistan and fight a jihad against the Russians was not very successful. The traditional Sunni position on *jus ad bellum* was that jihad was justified for defensive purposes only—not for assaults on non-Muslims. Even the defense of Central Asian Muslim communities against Russian ambitions in the region was inspired as much by the Salafi "Afghan Arabs," as they were called, as by local Islamic groups in the beginning. In fact, the modern debate in Islam about raising an Islamic army to fight the enemies of Islam was greatly enhanced by the war in Afghanistan in the 1980s and early 1990s. Osama bin Laden was among the Salafi ideologues who advanced that debate. He was by no means alone in arguing for violent use of jihad against enemies. In this context we should recall that the CIA and other arms of the U.S. government were the main financial backers and weapons suppliers of Osama bin Laden in the ultimately successful jihad waged against the Soviet Union, whose defeat brought an end to the Soviet empire. Osama was our mercenary friend in the 1980s.

In a very informative analysis of the contemporary Salafi movement, Quintan Wiktorowicz shows that in addition to the jihadi (often called the *mujahidun* or mujahideen) wing of the Salafi movement, there is also a reformist wing.[21] Wiktorowicz argues that all branches of the Salafi movement believe that jihad must be waged against the enemies of Islam (the Soviet Union, the United States, the West). As a proponent of social movement theory, Wiktorowicz argues against the view that Osama bin Laden and other radical jihadi Salafis are, because of their beliefs and acts, somehow beyond the pale of Islam. His analysis of jihadi Salafis stresses the religious texts and interpretive rules that jihadi Salafis share with other Muslims. He shows that the reformist mujahideen believe, however, that the Islamic world is too fictionalized and too disorganized to mount a successful global struggle against the forces of secularism, the Western powers, and global capitalism. The reformers advocate mounting a massive *da'wa* campaign of education about the true Islam and the purification of faith and practice. The Jama'at-e Islami groups in South Asia exemplify this nonviolent approach, through proselytism directed mainly toward the larger Muslim community. They argue that the path of violence by waging jihad against Islam's proven enemies at this time would be to exchange one evil for another of equal or greater weight, namely the self-destruction of the Muslim *umma*, the community of Muslim believers.

The jihadi branch of the Salafi movement claims, as did the assassins of late Egyptian president Anwar al-Sadat, that jihad, indeed militant jihad, has become a neglected Islamic duty in modern times. Moreover, they argue that jihad or armed struggle, overtly or covertly, falls to each individual to perform. Most Muslim jurists have regarded jihad as combat to be a *fard kifaya*, that is, a duty that the community as a whole, but not each and every Muslim, must fulfill in combat against Islam's enemies. The jihadi Salafis have reinterpreted it as a *fard 'ayn*, a duty that falls to each individual to fulfill in some significant way. In this, they are tilting against the much larger Sunni and Shi'i legal tradition. Historically and politically, support for the use of violence in jihad has evolved, especially in the past few decades, when regimes in Egypt, Algeria, and elsewhere have taken violent, repressive action against nonviolent Islamic reform movements. The argument, then, is an inter-Islamic one, based on a common set of authoritative texts and a shared history of disputes about how to interpret those texts.

Conclusion

In a recent speech in Washington, D.C., journalist Cokie Roberts warned that reporters who raise critical questions about U.S. foreign policy are increasingly under fire by the huge shadow cast over them by the Patriot Act, signed on October 26, 2001, by President Bush. She urged her fellow journalists to insist to those who questioned their patriotism that asking critical questions, especially in times of national crisis, is a form of patriotism that is guaranteed by the Constitution. It is what good journalists do to help maintain an informed electorate and to encourage national leaders to be responsible and answerable to those who elected them. These are times when students and scholars should heed the same message. It is important to challenge the mindless attacks on Islam and on those who teach about Islamic history and culture, and especially on those colleagues and students and their families who are Muslim. It is especially incumbent upon us to regard very critically the claims made about Islam and Muslim faith communities. Ideologically and theologically inspired misrepresentations are particularly harmful and dangerous at this moment in time, when two United States–led wars are perceived throughout the Muslim world as being waged against Muslims. Muslims in America—most of whom are American citizens—suffer discrimination and humiliation from law enforcement agencies and neighbors, in schoolyards, and also from the still sadly influential pronouncements of religious spokespersons from the Christian right, such as Franklin Graham and Pat Robertson, who declare Muslims to be heathen and who demand the opportunity to follow U.S. troops to Afghanistan and Iraq to proselytize in the name of a fundamentalist evangelical form of Protestantism.

The responsibility of scholars and students that I speak of also requires us to expose and analyze the conflicts among Muslims, in their historical development and in their modern particularities. That some Muslims called Salafis and Wahhabis have urged Muslims to conduct jihad against non-Muslims also needs to be studied, analyzed, and explained. It certainly does not need to be condoned. I remind readers that the scholarly activity of explaining and interpreting religious phenomena, including violent acts done in the name of religion, is not morally equivalent to advocating violence.

I have tried to make the case that Wahhabism and the Salafi movement more broadly are engaged in considerable dispute within Islam—

among Muslim scholars and intellectuals as well as in communities where Salafi missionaries have sought to spread their interpretation of Islam. I have argued that the Salafi movement is complex and itself divided between those who advocate active combat with Muslim and non-Muslim enemies, and those who do not. Many Salafi Muslims are advocates of peace who nonetheless hold puritanical theological views. Those Muslims who actively support the Salafi movement, especially the jihadi branch, are estimated to be very small in number compared to the overall population of over one billion people who claim Islam as their faith. Other intellectual and social-movement trends in the contemporary Muslim world include groups that self-identify as liberal, progressive, modernist, and traditionalist.

Globalization, the Internet, and Saudi funds have helped the Salafi movements to grow and spread despite official condemnation of most of them by many orthodox Muslim leaders and institutions. Events liked the Afghan war, in both its Soviet and American phases, have also globalized the Salafi movement, drawing supporters and sympathizers from diverse countries and backgrounds. European colonialism, post-colonial political and cultural disintegration, and U.S. foreign policy are also a part of the story of why young Muslim males have turned to Salafi interpretations of Islam for religious and indeed modern identity.

A reconciliation of reformist and jihadi Salafi social movements, as well as the Salafi identity overall with mainstream Islamic groups, is something that Muslims will have to work out. Muslim intellectuals on both sides of these disputes are beginning to discuss their differences, using traditional religious as well as modern critical theory and philosophical discourse to stake out their positions. Many of these groups find common cause with non-Muslim religious and humanitarian groups on some matters more readily than with fellow Muslims. In this vastly more complex understanding of contemporary Islam, there is little ground on which to build a case for dividing the Islamic world into good and bad Muslims. These are social movements and interpretive communities that have had good and bad moments in recent history.

My point is not against our moral and democratic right to judge religious activities to be good or bad, criminal or civilized, justified or unjustified. Rather, my point is against making judgments about Islamic movements and actors before we know much about them, or understand them in the context of their own political histories and religious interpretive communities.

Notes

1. Edmund Burke III and Ira M. Lapidus, eds., *Islam, Politics and Social Movements* (Berkeley: University of California Press, 1988), p. 19.

2. Ibid., p. 18.

3. See, for example, Roxanne L. Euben, *Enemy in the Mirror: Islamic Fundamentalism and the Limits of Modern Rationalism, a Work of Comparative Political Theory* (Princeton: Princeton University Press, 1999).

4. Bruce B. Lawrence, *Shattering the Myth: Islam Beyond Violence* (Princeton: Princeton University Press, 1998).

5. John L. Esposito, *The Islamic Threat: Myth or Reality?* 3d ed. (New York: Oxford University Press, 1999).

6. "Clash of Civilizations or an Islamic Reformation?" A public lecture delivered at Emory University on September 11, 2002.

7. The following section was inspired by a paper by Bruce Lawrence, "Conjuring with Islam II," presented at the conference "Critical Issues in Islamic Studies" at Stanford University, May 2–3, 2002.

8. Fiachra Gibbons, "Naipaul Lets Rip at 'Banality' of Indian Women Writers," *Guardian*, February 22, 2002.

9. V.S. Naipaul, *Among the Believers: An Islamic Inquiry* (London: Andre Deutsch, 1981), and Naipaul, *Beyond Belief: Islamic Excursions Among Converted Peoples* (London: Little, Brown, 1998).

10. Francis Fukuyama, *The End of History and the Last Man* (New York: Free Press, 1992).

11. September 1990: 52–60.

12. Ibid, p. 60.

13. *What Went Wrong: Western Impact and Middle Eastern Response* (Oxford and New York: Oxford University Press, 2001).

14. John Kelsay, "Bosnia and the Muslim Critique of Modernity," in *Religion and Justice in the War over Bosnia*, ed. G. Scott Davis (New York and London: Routledge, 1996), p. 119.

15. See Mumtaz Ahmad, "Islamic Fundamentalism in South Asia: The Jamaat-I-Islami and the Tablighi Jamaat of South Asia," in *Fundamentalisms Observed*, eds. Martin E. Marty and R. Scott Appleby (Chicago and London: University of Chicago Press, 1991), pp. 464–68.

16. Sayyid Qutb, *Milestones* (Beirut: Holy Koran Publishing House, 1978), and in several subsequent English editions, most recently published by Kazi Publications, Chicago.

17. For a good assessment of the influence of IT globalization on Muslim social movements, see Peter G. Mandaville, "Reimagining the Ummah? Information Technology and the Changing Boundaries of Political Islam," in Ali Mohammadi, ed., *Islam Encountering Globalization* (London: RoutledgeCurzon, 2002), pp. 61–90.

18. Ibn Taymiyya's fourteenth-century assault on religious syncretism and non-Muslim innovations in Islamic spiritual life has been translated into English by Muhammad Umar Memon, *Ibn Taimiya's Struggle Against Popular Religion* (The Hague: Mouton, 1976).

19. A nuanced and well-documented discussion of ibn Hanbal and Hanbalism, as well as the Ash'arites and the distinction between them and the former, is found in Michael A. Cook, *Commanding Right and Forbidding Wrong in Islamic* (Cambridge: Cambridge University Press, 2000).

20. Related by personal communication from Dr. Hanaa Kilany, Emory University, November 2002.

21. Quintan Wiktorowicz, "The New Global Threat: Transnational Salafis and Jihad." (Available from the author: visit www.newswise.com/articles/2001/11/SALAFI.RHD.html [viewed February 23, 2003]).

Part II

Science and Reconciliation

Reconciling Trauma and the Self

The Role of Narrative in Coping with Sexual Abuse and Terrorism

Robyn Fivush

How do we speak about the unspeakable? When trauma occurs, how do we come to comprehend and narrate that experience and how does it change the way we understand who we are in the world? Trauma, by definition, is an overwhelming experience, an event that is unthinkable and senseless, one for which we have few defenses yet must defend against. Moreover, a traumatic event is not over once the experience itself comes to an end; rather, trauma lives on in our minds, playing itself out again and again as we attempt to comprehend what is, at core, beyond comprehension.

One of the most enduring consequences of experiencing trauma is what Janoff-Bulman[1] has called "shattered assumptions." Most of us are fortunate enough to grow up in a world in which we believe that we are safe, that people are not evil, and that, for the most part, we have some control over what happens to us. For those who experience trauma, these assumptions are shattered. After experiencing severe trauma, individuals can no longer assume a benevolent world. Expectations of personal safety and predictions about the future are drastically altered. One can no longer assume that "everything will be all right." Indeed, severe trauma often leads to expectations of continued distress and an inability to predict the future. This is certainly true in cases of individual trauma, and for many of us living in the aftermath of the terror attacks of 9/11, it is also true for those who have experienced collective trauma. Even for those who did not know anyone killed in the attacks, the events of 9/11 changed the world and assumptions about safety and security.

Two questions about the consequences of experiencing trauma are key. First, if trauma, by definition, is incomprehensible, then how do trauma survivors comprehend it? More specifically, how do trauma survivors come to remember and recount their experiences? Are survivors able to provide a coherent narrative of what occurred? And if so, does this matter? What is the relation between the coherence of a survivor's narrative and his/her ultimate ability to cope with the trauma? This leads to the second question: how does trauma change the way in which one sees oneself? If trauma shatters our assumptions about the world, then how might these shattered assumptions change the way in which we see ourselves and our place in the world? First, it is necessary to touch on some theory about relations between trauma and memory, focusing on the issue of narrative coherence. I will then turn to a discussion of two studies examining relations between narrative coherence and self-concept, one focusing on the individual trauma of childhood sexual abuse and the second focusing on the collective trauma of 9/11. Finally, I will discuss how trauma changes our sense of self and our place in the world, and the ways in which we struggle to reconcile trauma with a coherent sense of self and meaning in the world.

The relations between memory and trauma are complex and paradoxical. There are two competing common-sense beliefs about memory of trauma. On one hand, it is commonly assumed that trauma is so devastating, so life-changing, that it is recalled in all too vivid detail, as if it were burned into the brain. Indeed, William James[2] claimed that trauma left a "scar on the cerebral tissue." On the other hand, trauma is so overwhelming that we do not have the cognitive resources to process it, and therefore traumatic events are poorly recalled, perhaps even repressed or kept from mind as too threatening.[3] Perhaps not surprisingly, there is empirical support for both positions. Some individuals who experience trauma recall the event in vivid detail, whereas others claim to have no memories at all. Most intriguing, both of these subjective memory phenomena can coexist within the same individual, dynamically changing over time. Individuals who suffer from post-traumatic stress disorder (PTSD), a relatively common response to trauma, claim to have periods of vivid memory, more like reliving the event than simply recalling it, and other periods where the event is almost completely forgotten.[4] Recent neuropsychological evidence indicates that traumatic events are processed differently by the brain than nontraumatic events, and many of these differences seem to be related to differences in subsequent memory.[5]

The question arises as to whether it matters if and how we remember trauma. Perhaps it is better for trauma to remain unremembered and unexpressed. Yet the evidence seems to suggest not. More specifically, it matters not just whether we remember trauma, but *how* we remember it. There is accumulating evidence that more coherently organized narratives of stressful and traumatic events lead to better physical and mental health outcomes. In a programmatic series of empirical studies, Pennebaker and his associates[6] have demonstrated that the act of simply writing about a stressful event several times over a period of a few days is associated with better physical health even months later. More intriguing, there are specific aspects of narrative change over the retellings that are associated with better outcome. Individuals whose stories become more coherent, better organized in terms of causal and explanatory frameworks, and more emotionally integrated in terms of including both negative and positive emotions, show the best outcome. This effect has now been demonstrated in college students, army recruits, and middle-aged corporate executives, among many others. Further, even if the narratives are about mildly stressful events in the individual's everyday life, the effect still holds. This line of research has established that narrating about stressful experiences, especially in ways that help to create more coherent causal and emotional frameworks for understanding the events, facilitates coping even with everyday stressors.

Within the clinical community, there is also growing evidence that helping clients create coherent narratives of traumatic events is beneficial. Foa, Molnar, and Cashman[7] studied adult rape survivors for the first twelve months following the event. All of the women showed symptoms of post-traumatic stress disorder during the first one to three months following their attack. PTSD symptoms include nightmares, feelings of re-living or re-experiencing the trauma, intrusive thoughts, an inability to focus or concentrate, and bodily symptoms including insomnia, sweats, and irritability, among others. Women who had been raped were randomly assigned to one of two interventions—either desensitization therapy, in which they were taught relaxation and meditation techniques that allowed them to think about the trauma without decompensating, or narrative therapy, in which the women were asked to narrate in detail the attack, over and over and over with the therapist. The control group consisted of a third group of women who were asked to wait three months for therapy. Women's PTSD symptoms were then assessed at the end of the three-month therapy intervention or waiting period and again a year later. All women showed some improvement at both three months and a year, indicating that PTSD symptoms abate with time even without intervention. But women in the desensitization group showed greater improvement over the first three months than women in the control group, and women in the narrative group showed even greater abatement of symptoms than women in the desensitization group. Most important, a year later, women who had been in narrative therapy still showed the least symptomotology. Again, the greatest improvement even within the narrative therapy group was associated with the ability to construct a more coherent narrative. Thus, there is good evidence that individuals who are able to construct more coherent narratives about stressful and traumatic events in their lives show better outcomes than those who are not.

Why are more coherent narratives associated with better coping? This is still an open question, and different theorists have proposed the existence of different mechanisms. As with all complex phenomena, the ultimate answer will surely be an interaction of multiple factors, but here I focus on relations between coherence, coping, and self-concept. One reason that coherent narratives lead to better coping is that coherent narratives provide us with a framework for understanding the traumatic event, which in turn allows us to integrate the trauma with self-understanding. Returning to the idea of shattered assumptions, trauma not only shatters assumptions about the world but also about the self. By throwing the individual into an unpredictable, malignant world, trauma destroys the sense of self-integrity. If individuals have no control, if they cannot explain what has happened, then they lose a sense of themselves as efficacious beings acting in a predictable world. Just as trauma throws the world into turmoil, so, too, does it throw the self into turmoil. In creating coherence out of this chaos, individuals regain control over both the world and the self. More specifically, from this perspective, individuals who are unable to create coherent accounts of trauma would be unable to integrate the trauma into their self-concept, leading to dissociation. In contrast, those individuals who are better able to create coherent accounts of traumatic incidents would thus be able to reconcile trauma with their sense of who they are in the world.

We explored this issue in an in-depth interview study with adult women who experienced severe childhood sexual abuse.[8] Childhood sexual abuse is a particularly interesting type of trauma from a theoretical perspective for several reasons. First, it occurs early in development, while the individual is still forming her/his sense of the world. What kind of world view would a child construct if exposed to trauma as a "normal" experience? Related to this, childhood sexual abuse is most often a recurring event. Predictions about the world are based on events that are recurring and familiar. These are the events that give the most information about how the world works. In this case, assumptions are being formed rather than shattered.[9] Finally, the vast majority of sexual abuse is perpetrated by someone the child knows, often a family member. Thus childhood sexual abuse involves both physical and emotional trauma. Not only is it difficult for the child to understand the sexual acts themselves and place them in an appropriate context, sexual abuse is even more traumatic because of the emotional betrayal by a loved and trusted elder.[10] Finally, memory of childhood sexual abuse is quite variable.[11] Whereas some women claim to remember their abusive experiences in great detail with no loss of memory over time, others claim to forget either all or some of their abusive experiences for periods of time. The issue of so-called "recovered" memories is complex, but suffice it to say here that there is good evidence that women who claim to have forgotten experiences of childhood sexual abuse and to have then subsequently remembered these experiences are just as likely to have corroborative evidence for their abuse as women who have had continuous memories—and most women who claim to have been sexually abused are able to provide at least some corroborative evidence.[12]

In this study, we interviewed twelve women between the ages of twenty-one and seventy-five who had experienced severe and chronic sexual abuse during childhood. Table 1 shows the characteristics of the sample. As can be seen, all twelve women were abused by a close family member. Age at onset of abuse varies from preschool to preteen; most of the women experienced abuse for at least two years, and all experienced penetration, so this represents a severely abused sample. Not surprising in a sample of this severity, three-quarters of the women experienced additional sexual abuse either in childhood or adulthood, and just over half were also otherwise physically abused. It is important to point out that all of the women had been in therapy at some point. Although none of them had recovered memories of abuse while in therapy, some had regained access to memories prior to therapy. The interviews were semi-structured, beginning with an open-ended question asking women to "Tell me everything you remember about your abusive experiences." After narrating their abuse experiences, the women

Table 1

Characteristics of the Sample

Participant number	Age at onset of abuse	Perpetrator	Other abuse		Abuse memory
			Physical	Sexual	
2	1 yr.	grandfather	yes	yes	recovered
3	2 yrs.	grandmother	no	no	recovered
4	2 yrs.	father	no	yes	recovered
7	5 yrs.	brother	yes	yes	continuous
9	5–6 yrs.	uncle	yes	yes	recovered
11	5 yrs.	brother	yes	yes	continuous
5	6–7 yrs.	father	yes	no	continuous
1	8 yrs.	father	yes	yes	continuous
6	8 yrs.	grandfather	no	no	recovered
8	10 yrs.	uncle	yes	no	continuous
10	12 yrs.	brother-in-law	yes	no	continuous
12	12 yrs.	stepfather	yes	yes	recovered

were asked a series of questions about their experiences of remembering and forgetting the abuse. No questions focused explicitly on their self-concept.

Analyses focused on three main aspects of the interviews: (1) Did women give coherent accounts of their abusive experiences? (2) Did women claim to have continuous or recovered memories of the abuse? and (3) How did women express their self-concept in these interviews?

First, coherence. Not surprisingly, there were individual differences in how coherently women reported their experiences. Half of the women gave a clear, concise, and coherent account of what had happened to them, and half of the women gave incoherent, fragmentary accounts of what had occurred. To illustrate, here is the response of one woman to the initial question. This woman was abused by her father beginning about age six, and this narrated episode is the beginning of what was a much longer account:

> My earliest memory that I can really identify as a specific instance was when I was about six, six or seven. And, uh, my family had gone to the Boys Scout Camp that my father was a Boy Scout executive and he had actually been the kingpin in getting this camp built. And at the end of the camping season, the Boy Scout leaders and their families had a little scouting experience, camping experience to use up all the staples and close the camp and so forth. And one day we took, there were a large group of us, a large group of parents and children that took a hike out in the shrub, umm, scrub brush. You don't get a lot of forest or anything in that part of

the state that I was, uh, and, uh, the others went one way and my dad and I went another. And I remember we ended up lying down in the dirt. Actually I was afraid the ants would get on me, while he, uh, fondled me and had me fondle him. And I don't know whether that was the first incident but I remember that I think, because of the peculiar circumstances that surrounded it, the fact that we were out in brush country, and, uh, but from then on I can remember several things specifically.

This is a clear story, providing information about the setting, the people, and the actions, as well as what she was thinking and feeling during the event. This woman then goes on to give several more very specific episodes of abuse, all of which were clear and coherent. Contrast this with another woman who was also abused by her father. She has difficulty reporting a clear incident, moves back and forth in time, and is unable to paint a coherent picture:

Well, I'm 48 now and probably when I was about 46, something like that, umm, and stuff I've been going through, umm, up until I was about 46, I remembered, umm, my dad, uh, when my mom was gone and all the other kids were gone, had me sleep in his room and wanted me to, I guess you'd say give him a hand job, or, sounds so funny. Um, anyways, so I was at that time, I was, I would take a wild guess, I don't know. Maybe 5 or 6 years old. And then, after I've been going through this stuff, it's like, uh, remembering all this stuff that was there that you just, I think you're lucky to block it out a lot of times but, uh, just as a baby, baby, I mean very small, I remember my dad, you know, molesting me. Uh, having intercourse with me and I was, I don't know, as far as I can remember, I get pieces that might have been earlier, but, uh, I don't know, as young as like two to three years old. So I'm not even sure if I've got all the pieces yet.

This woman continues to move back and forth in time, giving snippets of details here and there with no clear connections among incidents and no clear narrative line. Did narrative coherence bear any relation to other aspects of the women's memories?

Women were asked if they had always remembered the abuse, if they always remembered it in as much detail, and did they ever actively try to forget their abusive experiences, among other questions. Here the women fell into three groups. The first group of three women, described in Table 2, claimed they had always recalled the abuse and always recalled it in as much detail. The second group, also of three women, also claimed to have always remembered the abuse, but the level of detail differed at

Table 2

Subjective Memory Experiences

Group I: Continuous memories; no loss of details

Participant	Abuser	Memory Experience
5	father	I certainly never forgot it.
7	brother	There's not a time I've ever forgotten.
11	brother	I remembered it all along.

Group II: Continuous memories; differing levels of detail

Participant	Abuser	Memory Experience
1	father	. . . a lot of this has resurfaced.
8	uncle	I don't remember a lot of the details. . . . I fight to remember things.
10	brother-in-law	Since I've started talking about it, I've remembered more.

Group III: Recovered memories

Participant	Abuser	Memory Experience
2	uncle	When it came out all of a sudden, I just started crying.
3	grandmother	Basically my [memory] was one flashback that happened 12 years ago.
4	father	I had just completely forgotten.
6	grandfather	It's resurfaced twice that I know of or that I remember . . . sometimes I wouldn't remember it for years.
9	grandfather	I lost memory . . . until I was in my 20s and it all came to me it seemed in kind of a rush.
12	stepfather	I would totally forget about it. . . . In my early 20s I became aware.

different times. Finally, the third group of six women claimed that there was a time when they did not recall their abuse. These women would be categorized as having "recovered" memories. However, when questioned further about their memory experiences, five of the six women claimed that they did not totally forget the abuse. Most of these women claimed that they sort of always knew the abuse had occurred but that they had actively tried to forget it, to block it from their minds. In a very real sense, these women were struggling with remembering and not remembering, with knowing and not knowing that the abuse had occurred, in contrast to the women in the first two groups who had had continuous memories.

Intriguingly, of the six women who claimed to have continuous memories, five gave a coherent narrative of the abuse. In contrast, of the six women who claimed to have forgotten the abuse for a period of time, five gave incoherent, fragmented responses when narrating their abuse. So it seems that women who actively try to forget their abusive experiences are reasonably successful at it. They report having less continuous memories, and the memories themselves seem more fragmented. What are the consequences of this coping strategy for self-concept?

Although we did not ask any specific questions about self-concept, all of the women spontaneously talked about the relation between their abuse experiences and their self-understanding, although in very different ways, as described in Table 3 in this chapter. Three of the women expressed a dissociated self-concept. They dealt with their abusive histories by blocking them out of awareness, by not thinking about it, and essentially not dealing with it. Not surprisingly, all three of these women claimed to have no memory of the abuse for a period of time. They also provided incoherent, fragmentary narratives. So these women simply have not worked toward integrating their early abuse experiences with their current understanding of self in the world.

Two women expressed continuing emotional turmoil surrounding the abuse. These were the only two women in the sample who were still dealing with extreme feelings of anger, as the quotes in the Table indicate, which suggests that they still feel victimized by the abuse. These two women also claimed to have forgotten about the abuse for a period of time, and both gave incoherent narratives. In contrast to the women who dissociate from the abuse, these women continue to identity with the abuse all too well; they are still unable to resolve the emotional impact of their histories.

Finally, seven of the women expressed a sense of reconciliation with their traumatic past. Although these women were clear that the abuse had greatly affected their lives in negative ways, they had managed to come to terms with their history and accept the trauma as part of who they are, as their quotes illustrate. Importantly, two of these women clearly expressed dissociative tendencies. They indicated that at some point they had dissociated their abusive experiences from conscious awareness. However, in contrast to the women who were still expressing dissociation in the present, these women, at some point, confronted their histories. Reconciliation is expressed in several ways: as trying to analyze

Table 3

Abuse and Self-Concept

Self as Dissociated

#2
That was the very beginning of my learning how to take myself away from my body.
I can be a watcher anytime I want to be. So they can't hurt me anymore. Nothing
can hurt me anymore. It doesn't matter what happens to my body because they
can't hurt me.

I've got it pretty much taken care of because I'm familiar with all those different L___'s
with all the different histories. And that's all it is, history . . . that was a different person
or a different time . . . there is no use in thinking about that kind of stuff.

#3
I heard about sexual abuse but I didn't really associate it with me. . . . It was like it
went in and it went out and I didn't want to approach it.

I still can't separate the good parts from the negative, to sit there and get angry,
umm, and, I, there are a lot of things I just have not learned . . . umm, there is a major
block of emotional growth that never happened that I'm having to learn now.

#4
It's still hard for me to accept . . . there are occasions, even, I guess it's called denial,
even knowing all of it. Once in a while, I mean, it goes through my head, like, oh, you
know I must be nuts or I'm making all this up. I mean fathers, how could they do this?

I just kind of, you know, put it on the back burner. And there's, you're not going to get,
I mean, what, again, what are your options? So you might as well just shut up and try
to forget it.

Self as Victim

#6
. . . there's a lot of anger. There's a lot of sadness, just that it happened, like why did
it have to happen to me? Um. Why does it have to happen to anybody but why does
it have to happen to me?

#12
I'm angry. I'm very angry. My anger was brought to the forefront. But this is like 30,
well, a little less than 30, 25 years I'd say later, and you know, it's like I've gone
through this and I'm trying to work it out.

I'm just looking for relief.

Self as Reconciled

#1
I feel like I am getting more able to make decisions. . . . I feel like I must have some
sort of survival skills.

#5
I confronted my dad after mother died. And I told him, I said, you know, if I could understand why you did this, what made you do it, uh, maybe I could get rid of this lump in my stomach. . . . And I said, well, I guess I forgive you but I can't forget it. I said, I have a certain amount of love for you because you're my father. But I don't like you at all.

I've only tried to understand. And I've overanalyzed everything.

#7
You try to get involved in other things and just say the past is the past and we have to go on, you know. . . . I gotta quit dwelling on the past. You can't, you can't hold on. It's not going to do any good. I call it starting to grow. . . Now I feel like I'm growing more and more everyday. I'm learning more and more. Finally growing old and learning to put things in perspective and put things in the past that belong in the past. Go for the future.

#8
I had to figure out why it was so hard for me to trust. . . . And I think that's one of the things that's just part of me now.

Now I know that it was completely his fault . . . individuals should exercise common sense and respect the rights of children.

#9
I don't go to that place in my head where I'm being abused.

I remember the shame and this view of there being something wrong with me. . . . On the other hand, there's a great deal of relief because knowing, learning about sexual abuse as a child and understanding that that's what happened to me gives me a framework for making sense out of a lot of my early years, and, and, some of the things that, some of the self-image problems that I had, some of the acting out I did, some of my own struggles. . . .

I carry it around with me as part of my day. . . . I'm much more accepting of it. I don't respond with a great deal of, oh my god, uh, this happened, or, it's really like a matter of my history . . . I mean, it's one of those biographical facts about me. That's just part of who I am.

#10
And what I did with it was, I would totally forget about it. I mean I would internalize it and dissociate it basically. And so it was like it never happened.

Now there's been some healing. I've been in recovery eight years, so, you know, the alcohol was used a lot during the twenties to cover up a lot of feelings, I mean a lot, I was abusing myself more than he could ever have abused me. I've had, fortunately, a lot of healing in my life. . . Then underneath all this is, do I forgive him? I have to for my own health.

#11
I grew up through my teenage years thinking I was bad . . . that I had this hidden badness side to me, umm, and now, you know, I don't throw it away anymore. . . . I'm more, like, I definitely put the responsibility on him for it.

and comprehend what happened, as forgiving the abuser, as accepting the abuse as part of who one is but not totally self-defining, and, perhaps most poignantly, as forgiving oneself. Six of these women had continuous, coherent memories.

These patterns suggest that the ways in which one copes with trauma affect both memory and self. Women who push their abusive experiences out of conscious awareness, who cope by splitting part of their experiences off from their life history, have a more fragmented memory of what occurred. Some of these women continue to split their memories from their selves and express a dissociated sense of self; they simply try to ignore what has happened. Other women embrace their abusive histories almost too tightly, still expressing raw emotion. Both of these strategies seem to lead to periods of not remembering the abuse, perhaps because it is still too emotionally difficult. In contrast, some women seem to be able to come to terms with their experiences. They clearly do not deny the negative effects their histories have had on their lives, but they seem better able to accept these experiences as part of who they are. These women seem to have thought about, analyzed, processed their experiences to a greater extent. And, indeed, they claim to have continuous memories, and their narratives are quite coherent.

It must be emphasized that these women were all survivors in a very real sense. They had horrific childhood experiences yet were all leading productive adult lives. But the ways in which they survived differed. For some women, survival necessitated cutting off a part of oneself, perhaps permanently. For others, the raw emotional response to their history may never be resolved. Yet about half of these women were able to somehow come to terms with their experiences. Perhaps by creating more coherent narratives that provided some kind of explanatory framework, these women managed to reconcile trauma with self-understanding.

Experiencing childhood sexual abuse at the hands of a loved and trusted adult is quite likely at the extreme of traumatic events. Because it occurs in childhood when concepts of self and the world are being formed, it would totally disrupt normal developmental processes, leading to a view of the self as victim or, perhaps even worse, as guilty conspirator, and the world as unsafe and unforgiving. Moreover, childhood sexual abuse is totally isolating. It occurs in private, and the child is usually threatened or otherwise cajoled into not telling anyone what is happening. Even when children do disclose the abuse, they are most often not believed,[13] escalating their sense of unreality and lack of safety. Quite likely, these factors lead to the severity of difficulties these women face in constructing a coherent sense of the experiences and of themselves.

From Private to Public Trauma

But what about more public trauma? How do we make sense of traumatic events that occur in the open, events that are acknowledged and mourned? Unfortunately, the events of the last few years have provided a natural experiment. The terror attacks of 9/11 were traumatic on many levels, but perhaps most poignantly, they established American vulnerability. In addition to the thousands who were killed in the attacks, there was the ongoing fear of not being able to predict or prevent additional attacks. As many commentators pointed out, it was the first time in half a century that Americans were killed on their own ground, and, different from previous attacks such as Pearl Harbor, the first time that attacks focused on everyday civilians. How can we live in a world in which we are not safe leaving our house in the morning?

A colleague and I are examining how Emory undergraduates are coping with the events of 9/11 in an ongoing diary intervention study.[14] We were particularly interested in examining college students because this is a time in their lives when individuals are struggling with issues of identity and self-concept.[15] How might a national tragedy of this scope influence students' ongoing dialogue with themselves about who they are in the world and how they want to structure their lives? Eighty-five undergraduates participated in the larger project, which explores long-term relations among the diaries and multiple measures of anxiety, depression, and coping. Approximately one month after 9/11, students were asked to keep a diary; they were instructed to write about their thoughts and emotions about 9/11 for approximately twenty minutes a day for five consecutive days. By chance, fourteen of the students knew someone who was killed in the World Trade Center collapse. Thus these students faced both personal and collective trauma. Here I focus on a qualitative analysis of two of these students' diaries.

The first diary is from a male student who knew two people killed in the World Trade Center—his childhood Little League coach, whose son he is still friends with, and an adult male neighbor. He does not mention these deaths in his first diary entry, but rather focuses on his fears about his family on that day:

When I first heard about the attack I was in PE class. When I saw the news I was both scared and confused. I could not believe that a plane had just crashed into the World trade center. Two thoughts came into my mind: one was that my father lives in the city and second that friends of mine have brothers and family members who actually work in the building. I tried to call my Dad and could not get through. . . . [He narrates about returning to his dorm room, still unable to make contact by phone, and then going online.] The emotions that were going through me were unmatched. I was a combined terrified, upset, angry, and on top of that I was filled with nausea. I thought to myself, how and why would anyone possibly do this? As the expected death counts increased I became disgusted. . . . [he comments on how crazy terrorists are.] Sometimes I think to myself on how I would have reacted if I had been on the plane while it was under the control of the terrorists. I hope to think that I would be the hero and attempt to stop what was going on but one can never know unless he were in that situation. Again, I think to myself that I would devise a plan and retake the plane and lead everyone to safety.

We see in this excerpt, first, the high level of emotional intensity this individual faced that day. The disbelief, the fear for loved ones, the terror of not being able to make contact. But he ends on an interesting note. His way of coping at this point is to create a fantasy resolution in which he would have been able to save the day. This is both soothing to one's sense of fear as well as bolstering to one's sense of self as effective and safe in the world. On the second and third day of writing, he talks about hearing the news of the deaths of those he knew. Again, he comments about the devastation. In writing about his friend's father's death, he states, "I cannot begin to imagine how I would feel if these events had occurred to me," yet at the same time minimizes the event by writing "but I have to say from an outsider's point of view that he just has to get on with it and live on." So again we see the tensions between the raw emotion and the need to resolve the emotion quickly. On days three and four the student continues to express anger and resentment at the terrorists as well as at the government that did nothing to stop the attacks. Yet on day five of writing, we see a sudden shift:

Because of all that occurred I view myself as a changed person. I am now more tentative about situations and I really do appreciate more what I have and my family's health. Again, I do not know what I would do if I were in [the friend's name] shoes. I also changed in that I am trying to lessen my temper. Sometimes I have the problem of taking not so important issues very seriously. I have realized that most things are not that important to argue over and getting into arguments can be easily avoided. Something else that has changed is my plans for the future. I am going to try to create a better me, not only with arguing but with many of my known flaws. . . . [He narrates about reading how Nostradamus had predicted this event.] My concluding thoughts on my accounts goes as follows: I have a continuous feeling of sadness and grief when I think of all the people who were killed, especially those I knew personally. I have a hatred and personal anger against all of who were involved in the massacre. I think to myself that I would like to personally get involved and fight if called to do so but then I think of my family and other important things that I would be missing.

For the first time, this individual is now confronting how this event has shaped and will shape his understanding of self. These events have caused him to reflect on his own behavior and beliefs about the world. But he still ends on a type of fantasy resolution similar to the first entry —one of revenge against the terrorists. Still, he now tempers this with the awareness that this would be a very difficult and arduous personal decision, thus reflecting an increasing ability to consider the complexities of the situation. Although he continues to express deep and abiding negative emotion, he ends his narrative looking forward to a positive future.

A different construction of the event emerges from the diary of a female student. Her first entry begins:

My good friend's mom died in the plane that hit the first tower. When I heard that awful news I could not control my absolute sadness and unyielding tears. I was already beside myself because I had been watching the news vigilantly for the first three days before I talked to my friend. . . . [She reports how she went to school in New York City for a semester.] When I saw the World Trade Center towers being taken away from me and my country I was immediately and permanently disheartened. I do not know how my friend got through the loss of her mother. I do not know.

As with the first diarist, this individual also expresses great emotion, but in contrast, she focuses on sadness and grief, not anger, and she is unable to resolve any of the adverse effects. It simply is. On day two, she expresses deep depression and even suicidal ideation: "My emotions about how to cope fluctuate from day to day. Once, right after the attacks, I sat in my room and cried. I did not see the point in letting my life go on when so many lives had just ended." On day three she states, "I do not expect these feelings to ever go away" and reports on a nightmare that she cannot shake from her consciousness. She ends this entry with "How can I go on with my everyday activities? How can I? But I do. I have to." Her fifth diary entry was on Veterans Day and the day a plane crashed flying out of LaGuardia airport due to engine failure. She writes:

> I try not to worry. Yesterday was the two-month anniversary and everything is still ok. I know my dad is flying today but that is ok because security is so high now . . . and I see on the news that another plane has crashed. I panic. I get frenzied. But it was not terrorists, it was not. It was the plane, they lost an engine. Somehow I am not consoled, not comforted. Where is my dad? Where is my mom? I call collect and no one is there. I start to cry. I call my nana. She says that it is ok, she doubts my dad is going to fly now, it is ok. I still cannot reach him. I cannot stand this feeling. . . . [She narrates an incident about a friend of hers trying to call someone after 9/11 and how afraid she is now of flying.] But I cannot live in this manner. People tell me I cannot live in fear. My nana says, "live for today, you cannot be scared." I believe her. It is fine. I am going to call my dad now.

In contrast to the first diarist, this individual shows no evidence of being able to resolve the sadness and fear, nor does she move into any kind of self-reflection. Her only self-referenced comments are about having to go on even though she does not see how she can. The affect is raw and almost debilitated. The anxiety is palpable.

Thus we see similar themes across narratives about childhood sexual abuse and the terror attacks of 9/11. In both cases, some individuals use the traumatic experience as the ground from which self-reflection and self-awareness will grow. Trauma redefines self, but not always in a negative way. The idea of "post-traumatic growth" is gaining acceptance in the literature in order to explain how some traumatized individuals are able to integrate trauma into a more complex, more self-reflective, and perhaps stronger sense of self in the world.[16] This is not to argue that the trauma itself ever becomes a positive experience, but rather that one is able to use this devastation to reconsider who one is and how one should live in the world, to reconcile trauma with one's evolving sense of self and the world. In contrast, some individuals seem less able to move beyond the raw emotional experience.

For them, trauma has also redefined self and world but no positive growth is evident; no reconciliation is possible. Instead, for these individuals, trauma diminishes who they are; it takes something away from the self rather than allowing self to grow. In both cases, trauma alters one's relationship to the world, but in the former case, it creates a challenge to be mastered while in the latter case it creates a barrier to integration and connection.

But we must be very clear what we mean by reconciliation. There may be some acts that are existentially unforgivable. Reconciliation does not necessarily mean forgiveness, or even understanding. Rather, reconciliation may be the simple acceptance that what happened cannot be changed. One must simply learn how to live with it, and with oneself, in a changed world.

Notes

1. R. Janoff-Bulman, *Shattered Assumptions* (New York: Free Press, 1992).

2. W. James, *The Principles of Psychology* (New York: Dover, 1890).

3. S. Freud, *A General Introduction to Psychoanalysis* (New York: Pocket Books, 1953 [1924]).

4. D. Brown, A.W. Scheflin, and C.L. Whitfield, "Recovered Memories: The Current Weight of the Evidence in Science and the Courts," *Journal of Psychiatry and Law* 27 (1999): 5–156.

5. B.A. Van der Kolk, J.A. Burbridge, and J. Suzuki, "The Psychobiology of Traumatic Memory: Clinical Implications of Neuroimaging Studies." In *Psychobiology of Posttraumatic Stress Disorder*, ed. R. Yehuda and A.C. McFarlane. *Annals of the New York Academy of Sciences* 821 (1997): 99–113.

6. J.W. Pennebaker, *Opening Up* (New York: Guilford, 1997).

7. E.B. Foa, C. Molnar, and L. Cashman, "Change in Rape Narratives During Exposure Therapy for Posttraumatic Stress Disorder," *Journal of Traumatic Stress* 8 (1995): 675–690.

8. R. Fivush and V. Edwards, "Remembering and Forgetting Childhood Sexual Abuse," in press, *Journal of Childhood Sexual Abuse*.

9. R. Fivush, "Scripts, schemas and trauma." In *Essays in Honor of Jean Mandler*, ed. N. Stein, P. Bauer, and M. Rabinowitz (Mahwah, NJ: Erlbaum, 2002).

10. J. Freyd, *Betrayal Trauma: The Logic of Forgetting Childhood Abuse* (Cambridge, MA: Harvard University Press, 1996).

11. C.R. Brewin and B. Andrews, "Recovered Memories of Trauma: Phenomenology and Cognitive Mechanisms," *Clinical Psychology Review* 18 (1998): 949–970. See also K. Pezdek and W. Banks, *The Recovered Memory Debate* (New York: Academic Press, 1996).

12. C.R. Brewin and B. Andrews, "Recovered Memories of Trauma: Phenomenology and Cognitive Mechanisms," *Clinical Psychology Review* 18 (1998): 949–970. See also D. Brown, A.W. Scheflin, and C.L. Whitfield, "Recovered Memories:

The Current Weight of the Evidence in Science and the Courts," *Journal of Psychiatry and Law* 27 (1999): 5–156.

13. L. Butler, paper presented at the meetings of the International Society for Traumatic Stress Studies, San Antonio, TX, 1999.

14. R. Fivush and V. Edwards, "Coping with 9/11 Through Expressive Writing," *Applied Cognitive Psychology* 17 (2004): 1099–1112.

15. E. Erikson, *Youth and Identity Crisis* (New York: Norton, 1968).

16. R.G. Tedeschi, C.L. Park, and L.G. Calhoun, eds., *Posttraumatic Growth: Positive Change in the Aftermath of Crisis* (Mahwah, NJ: Erlbaum, 1998).

Reconciliation and the Craving for Revenge in Psychotherapy

Robert A. Paul

When President Bush promised he would "hunt down and kill" the people responsible for the terrorist attacks of September 11, he voiced an impulse that resonated both with many Americans and with one of the most ancient dynamics in human psychology: the craving for revenge. Using the same logic, spokesmen for al-Qaeda justified their attacks on the United States by saying "as you kill us, so we will kill you." While the desire to cause pain to those who have caused us pain seems to be directed outside the self, it also marks the site of a battle within the individual. Thus, one of the difficult tasks of psychotherapy involves attempts to reconcile a self divided by its own desires.

The process of psychotherapy often uncovers motives and impulses opposed to ones that patients consciously recognize as their own. Furthermore, many patients are not in any great rush to give up those goals and purposes that seem at first glance antithetical to their overall personalities. At the core of this struggle within the divided self are wishes, fantasies, and fears that are clung to with a passion and singleness of purpose at odds with the generally irresolute exterior presented by many patients. Woven around memories of episodes that may date back to early childhood, these fantasy formations—and the wishes and fears that characterize them—have been installed in the psyche as life projects meant to accomplish an important purpose. Sometimes, they aim to right some perceived wrong, obtain some long-cherished goal, or avoid some feared and anticipated personal catastrophe. But they always assume a form of thought that owes less to realistic analysis and rational planning than to the carrot of powerful impulse and the stick of dread, and the imaginative poiesis of a mind neither fully matured nor committed whole-heartedly to an acceptance of the necessities of social and physical real-ity. The particular fantasies I address in this essay are those that appear to be those built around the ever-postponed hope of settling scores. It is these that must be either abandoned or modified if inner reconciliation, and with it reconciliation with what is perceived as an inimical social milieu, is to be achieved through the psychological self-righting made possible in a successful psychotherapeutic treatment.

American society is one that, at least officially, operates under a zero-tolerance rule for the exercise of physical violence. There are no accept-able circumstances under which one person can legitimately do bodily harm to another, other than those authorized by a state agency, such as in war, capital punishment, or self-defense from violent acts. Even in these cases, the identity of the victim and the circumstances of the in-jury are strictly regulated and by no means a matter of personal choice. This does not mean, however, that wishes to do harm are absent from our imaginations. Certainly, they are plentiful and widespread and have no legitimate outlet in action in the ordinary course of things. What, then, are we supposed to do about them?

Often, as the current phraseology goes, we just "get over it." By this I mean that however robust and imperative an urge to inflict harm on someone who has crossed us may be, mature people realize that life will go on if we resist the temptation to act impetuously, and eventu-ally the hostile urge subsides. But in some cases this does not happen. Once set in motion, the determination to get our man (or woman) can seem immune to the wearing away with time that we expect of other strong but troubling impulses. In these situations, what seems to take hold of the personality is a fantasy dominated by a thirst for revenge. Examples of this extreme type are readily found in literature, from Cain's murder of his brother Abel in the Bible to Captain Ahab's quest for vengeance against his aquatic nemesis in *Moby Dick*. The pleni-tude of revenge-driven narratives reflects the widespread nature of the craving for vengeance in the psyches of actual people, and it also col-ors the interpretation that many people bring to contemporary events. The war against Iraq by the administration of President George W. Bush, for example, has been interpreted by some as an intergenerational revenge play, a kind of sequel to his father's battle against the same enemy. The current President Bush has been quoted as saying that one motive for the war is revenge for the Iraqi leader's alleged attempt to assassinate Bush Senior, and journalists and commentators can readily perceive in President Bush's threats against Saddam Hussein a quest to vindicate his father's failure to depose Saddam precisely because this story line of vengeance is always at our mental fingertips. The important question is, why is this the case?

The Anthropological Roots of the Revenge Fantasy

What is revenge, really, and why is it sometimes capable of motivating us beyond the bounds of reason, morality, and even self-preservation? As a psychologist and anthropologist, it is my view that there is probably an evolved, species-specific human propensity to form an abstract representation of what is done to one, and then to be able to picture its reversal. Such an ability would seem to be basic to the principle underlying the most elementary forms of human social organization—those depending on gift exchange and reciprocity. Social integration relies on our being able to tell when we are owed something, or when we are in someone's debt, and to direct our actions accordingly. To carry this off, we can picture a deed such as "Person A was nice to me" or "Person A gave me this much meat," and then we can, in thought, reverse it into such formulations as "I am nice to Person A" or "I give Person A the same amount of meat." The formal considerations of mathematical game theory, the theories of evolutionary psychology, the great sociological formulations of Marcel Mauss and Claude Levi-Strauss, and the psychoanalytic theory of object relations all concur that human sociality can be boiled down to the core maxim shared by many of the great religions: do as you are (or would be) done by. This may be considered the elementary form of justice and social harmony—that the balance of debt and obligation be relatively equalized among partners in a cycle of reciprocal dyadic interactions.

Revenge is the negative version of this. If the principle of reciprocity and the internal cognitive calculations we all make to keep it working insist that if someone gives us a gift we ought to give one back of equal or greater value; or, if my nuclear family gives yours a spouse to marry, sooner or later we should get one back; or, if I give you a certain amount of money, you are obligated to give me an object in trade of equivalent value; or, if I invite you to my daughter's wedding, I can expect to be invited to yours. So too goes the negative cognitive calculations: if you punch me in the nose, I ought to punch you back and hurt you as much as or more than you hurt me; or, if a member of your clan shoots a member of my clan, or gang, or whatever, we are entitled to take some shots at somebody in your clan, or gang, or whatever.

The emotional currency that fuels this system in an individual actor is what we refer to with such terms as pride, honor, prestige, and their opposites: shame, embarrassment, and humiliation. The person who fulfills her or his reciprocity obligations in a finely balanced network of social relations is entitled to feel a measure of socially recognized self-esteem. In a society dominated by a reciprocity ethic, this is equally true of the person who honors gift obligations and the person who fulfills a duty to avenge a slain kinsperson by killing an enemy clansman. The person who fails to meet such obligations suffers a fall in status, prestige, or recognition from peers that becomes mirrored in his or her own sense of failure and accompanying loss of honor, experienced as shame.

In minimal dyadic form, human social relations become zero-sum games over prestige, with winner-take-all being the rule. When two people play at this game, there will always be just a winner and a loser, unless perfect symmetry, or twinship, is maintained, or unless the two can fully identify with each other. When this dyadic structure of all-or-nothing, win/lose, either/or predominates, the only way to restore lost honor or to undo humiliation is to turn the tables in a way that restores the original status of things before the event that put one in the "one-down," losing position. All other values—personal safety, regard for others, material gain, social expectation, and law—fade into nothing in the face of the determination to undo humiliation and loss perceived to have come about at the hands of another. Hence we have the likes of Ahab's relentless pursuit of his nemesis, the whale who not only injured him but made him look bad by eluding his harpoons.

In societies without a strong centralized authority system, networks of reciprocity form the main social fabric. Justice requires the fulfillment of vengeance obligations, which are often codified in customary understandings that govern how they can be administered or averted by an adequate payment of ransom. But our society, as a state system with a strong central government, depends upon a monopoly of violence being held by the state itself through its institutions: the army, the courts, and the police. We citizens of such a society are asked to forgo the execution of retributive justice and believe instead in a depersonalized system of justice in which state bureaucrats maintain the public peace by settling our scores for us. We are taught from nursery school not to hit back if we are hit, that two wrongs do not make a right. And some religions offer a final piece of consolation with the hope that even if human justice fails to set things right, the Supreme Judge in heaven will, in the final hour, make sure that the overly prideful are humbled and the humiliated are redeemed in honor and glory. Note, however, that you can only have the idea of a supreme judge in heaven if you first have the institution of human judges on earth, and this institution only appears in human society with the rise of the state.

Notwithstanding the American official condemnation of the motive of revenge as a barbaric impulse that ought to be overcome by any civilized person or society, we have no more eliminated such ideation from ourselves or our culture than our zero-tolerance attitude toward violence has rendered us free of crime, or our Puritanism rid us of all traces of unregulated eroticism. We are a culture that can say in the same breath with "two wrongs do not make a right" things like "turnabout is fair play," "don't get mad, get even," and "make my day"—which is to say, "go ahead, do something to me (or to someone under my protection) that will justify my blowing you away; that would give me great pleasure indeed." We all recognize the narrative trope, so trite as to be a mere formula (but nonetheless *de rigueur* in a would-be box-office-smash action film) of the conflict between a lone hero of whom poetic justice requires an act of vengeance at odds with a state authority that is either too corrupt or too weak and namby-pamby to follow the code of honor and shame that we all understand. The enactment of this fantasy on the movie screen excites audiences for good reason.

The Psychological Roots of the Revenge Fantasy

Being a person—especially being a small, weak, uncoordinated person without any skill and therefore entirely dependent on the good will of someone better at life than you are—is an intrinsically humiliating experience, and we all go through it right at the beginning of life. Fortunately, nature has designed it so that this more able caretaker of ours is generally also a great admirer who is willing to grant us at least some measure of unconditional love and recognition of our personal dignity, even in our most awkward moments and despite our evident failings. If we can internalize a working model in our own psyches of such a "good-enough" mother, we are likely to be shielded from later feeling alone and at the mercy of a hostile and mocking world, at least most of the time.

But as psychotherapists we encounter in our patients a variety of personality types who feel that the wrongs done to them, and injustices to which they have been subjected, are sufficiently grievous that they cannot regain their damaged pride or self-esteem by the recognized avenues to ordinary achievement offered by society. For them, the size of the revenge they have coming to them is so enormous that reality cannot satisfy it—perhaps one reason that someone as driven by vindictive hate as Ahab needed to go after the biggest, meanest whale on earth, rather than just some human adversary. Such people feel "entitled," and what we mean by that is that they feel they have received an injury that entitles them to retribution of unlimited scale and of their own choosing, on whomever they choose and whenever it suits them. For such people, the ordinary rules of social life do not apply, since they are unable or unwilling to enter into the round of reciprocal relations. Until the injury to their self-esteem or honor has been avenged, they live in a state of suspended animation waiting for the opportunity that will fulfill the fantasy of satisfied honor through the revenge that they nurture. When they act out such fantasies, they can become terrorists.

Again, we find these psychological dynamics insightfully described in many works of literature. In his gem-like paper "The Exceptions," Freud cited Shakespeare's King Richard III as an example of just such a psychological constellation. For Freud, Richard felt justified in living a life of naked ambition and murderous inhumanity because his physical deformity had rendered him an object of ridicule and denied him the pleasures of ordinary courtship and love. For this slap that life had delivered, Richard felt himself to be an exception to every ordinary social and moral law, and entitled to take what he supposed the world now owed him by way of reparations. As Freud makes clear in his discussion of Kaiser Wilhelm's withered arm as a source of the latter's overweening ambition that brought Germany into the World War I, it was not the physical disability itself that was the problem or the goad, as Alfred Adler proposed with his theory of the "inferiority complex." Rather, Freud said, it was because his mother could not love a baby whose imperfection she regarded as a narcissistic blow to her own pride that Wilhelm, and presumably also Richard, felt his sense of absolute entitlement. A contemporary film, *My Left Foot*, offers a beautifully contrasting depiction of a mother who is perfectly capable of loving a baby with a far more severe physical disability than that of either Wilhelm or Richard, and of the very different effects this has on the child who, lacking control of three of his four limbs, becomes a successful writer holding the pen between the toes of his left foot and composes the deeply humane book upon which this film is based.

There are some patients who come to therapy or analysis with a prickly and querulous character, quick to anger and find fault, never satisfied, always able to make the therapist feel he or she is failing in empathy or understanding. These vindictive characters, whom we generally diagnose in the category of the narcissistic personality disorder, wear their sense of wronged victim entitled to retributive justice on their sleeves. They may seek to dominate and intimidate in any social encounter, including with the treating clinician, and their sensitivity to slights is as striking as their insensitivity to the feelings of others. Such people, generally harboring a deep fantasy of revenge against what they take to have been an inadequately loving parent (often a mother) who failed to safeguard their self-respect and dignity in childhood, may be remarkably adept at finding and creating ever new situations in which to reexperience their humiliation or to try to undo it by turning the tables on some unfortunate stand-in for the parent who is supposed to have humiliated or betrayed them. A man may, for example, constantly seduce women into perceiving him as a gentle and empathic lover, only to ditch them when they have fallen for him as a way of paying mother back for her perceived abandonment of her needy and dependent child long ago. Or a woman may go from one therapist to another, punishing each, as a substitutes for mother, by failing to improve, and leaving the therapy hurt, angry, and full of complaints about the inadequate understanding and care she received. These examples illustrate relatively straightforward cases of revenge as an regnant motivation, and often it is even understood as such by these patients, although they may feel incapable of doing anything about it or modifying it without external help—which, however, it is in the nature of their fantasy to feel bound to reject, devalue, or otherwise destroy. More likely, however, the man will genuinely feel that at first he is really attracted to each successive woman to be cast in his ongoing repetitive scenario, only to be really disappointed by the discovery of some previously unseen inadequacy; while the woman honestly thinks she is trying as hard as she can, and each new therapy that begins auspiciously runs aground on the failings of a wave of incompetent therapists.

While it is not too hard to discover the revenge motive in the unconscious fantasies guiding the lives of the overtly vindictive characters, many more people present themselves not with openly angry and vengeful agendas but rather with a variety of inhibitions and self-imposed limitations that keep them from performing up to their abilities or achieving their goals and plans. Upon deeper analysis, however, it very often emerges that a fantasy scenario of ultimate revenge for what is believed to be a deep humiliation resides at the heart of the psychology. The initial hurt may take many forms, from unempathic parenting, to perceived indifference or abandonment by a parent; jealousy over affection to which one feels entitled being showered on a sibling or on the parent's mate; envy of parental power, or of the prerogatives and attributes of the other sex; and many more. Here I should stress that I am not referring to people who have suffered actual traumatic injury or abuse at the hands of a parent, which Robyn Fivush addresses in another essay in this volume. At the core of the people I am describing—those with an exaggerated sense of entitlement—is a self-image of intrinsic unworthiness that has led to a failure to obtain the parental recognition and approval necessary to offset the humiliations of infantile dependency. This inner core is too vulnerable and shameful to be fully experienced, however, and so it is counteracted with a fantasy of being a winner rather than a loser, of being like the apparently omnipotent parent and making sure everyone he or she encounters comes away feeling devalued, through a reversal of the dyadic power relation. This self-image cannot be acted on either, however, because of the further logic of revenge: if it makes me this furious to have come off second best to you, you must surely feel the same way if I triumph over you, and then you will be out to get me just as I am now out to get you. Since this is a frightening thought, the whole grandiose defensive posture is also suppressed, and the person adopts an attitude toward the world that is designed not to achieve anything or draw anyone's admiration, for fear of seeming to be a victor and thereby reducing one's imaginary rival to humiliated loser thirsting for bloody retaliation. Hence the powerful commitment to inaction and inhibition—to mediocrity in work and failure in love—so often encountered in such persons. Their lives are "on hold," pending the enactment of the revenge scenario that is to clear their names, but is somehow always either indefinitely postponed, or else enacted on substitute victims, but always without satisfying the demand that only makes itself felt again sooner or later in the repetitive cycles so typical of neurotic characters.

Particularly striking in almost all such patients is the seemingly irrational, counterintuitive self-destructiveness and masochism at work with a kind of remorseless fury. There is not enough space here for a thorough investigation of this fascinating subject, but one aspect of it also reveals that it is a form of revenge against a parent perceived as having failed or betrayed one (as in the case of Kaiser Wilhelm or Richard III, cited earlier): Given the "all-or-nothing," zero-sum, winner-take-all nature of neurotic fantasy scenarios, all interactions are reduced to dyadic struggles in which one party loses and the other wins. It is equally intolerable to lose, which is humiliating, and to win, which only invites a dreaded retaliatory attack. The best that can be achieved, it seems, is a lose-lose situation, in which I make you suffer, but I suffer also, so as to forestall any need on your part to injure me, since I have already taken care of that for myself. Usually the patient knows very well that the most painful suffering she or he could inflict on a parent would be to suffer herself or himself, and fail to respond to any help that the parent might offer. This accomplishes the perversely desired goal, which is that both should feel unbearable anguish—the patient by suffering from neurosis, the parent from seeing a child suffering and feeling powerless to do anything about it.

This drama is enacted ubiquitously in therapy, where the patient maneuvers to achieve a situation of stasis in which the therapist is supposed to watch helplessly as the patient sinks into worse and worse shape. The revenge takes the reversed form of spite: "I wouldn't give you the satisfaction of helping me get better." Since any help or intervention of any kind from the therapist can be reinterpreted as a signal of the therapist's superior skill, mental health, professional credentials, or whatever, they must all be rejected, since otherwise they would stir up intolerable resentment of the therapist's having "won" the encounter by proving that he or she is better off than the patient.

I must stress that there is no notion implied here, though it may sound that way, of "blaming the mother," as a common complaint about psychotherapy or analysis has it. In the first place, one of the legitimate meanings of therapeutic neutrality is that we do not take a position pro or con about whether or not the person against whom the fantasy of revenge is directed really did anything bad enough to deserve it. Some people come unscathed through a set of experiences that sound hair-raising to us, while others develop deep narcissistic wounds from events that to us might seem minor. The object of the fantasy scenario is, in any event, a remembered and internalized image of a parent from years before, in early childhood. Often enough, a circumstance such as a hospitalization of the mother may be experienced as a profoundly disappointing abandonment by a child and demand retribution, even while the grown adult can see that there was no malice on the part of the mother. In other instances, there may be a genuinely bad temperamental match between mother and child, or a mother whose own personality prevents her from being able to adequately respond to or appreciate her child. Just as often, the malice that the child experiences coming at her from the parent is in fact her own rage and frustration turned around and attributed to the parent at whom it is in fact directed.

More importantly, however, there is absolutely no question of "blame" anywhere in this process. Blame is a concept belonging to the language of debt, obligation, guilt, punishment, shame, winners, losers, perpetrators, and victims from which it is our whole enterprise to liberate the patient's thinking, conscious and unconscious. Blaming the perpetrator, or blaming the victim, or blaming the parent or the child, is to collude in the either/or, zero-sum game of the dyadic unconscious scenario, which is precisely what is making the patient "sick." Psychotherapy is not a trial; it is a process of overcoming the compulsion to think in all-or-nothing terms about who wins or loses every possible human encounter or relationship.

How, then, is this transformation to be accomplished, especially in the face of the roadblocks to which I have referred already, including the patient's deep commitment to an impossible fantasy of ultimate vindication through a vengeful turning of the tables—doing to others as you have been done by—as well as the inability to accept help from another because of the repetition of humiliating dependency that it seems to entail?

Roots of Psychological Reconciliation

It seems clear that the project is one of forgiveness of, and reconciliation with, the person who is the object of the revenge fantasy. Yet this person is not a real person, but rather a fantasy figure composed of an accretion of memory, emotion, aggrandizement, and all sorts of other distortions. As often as not, by the time the patient seeks therapy, the parent at whom the original revenge fantasy was erected is dead or senile, or in any event a very changed person. The task, therefore, is reconciling not with a living person—though this can happen, and is certainly a good thing—but rather with a person who has become a presence in one's own mind, and usually in a part of one's mind over which one has little or no conscious control. Exhortations from the therapist to "forgive" are as futile as are the patients' repetitively made and broken promises to do so.

While there are many theories of psychoanalytic cure, probably the most elegant and certainly the most relevant for our present purposes is that developed by the school of Melanie Klein. According to Klein, negative feelings that arise between the child and its mother are initially handled by a fantasy of splitting: the child assumes that care and nurture are delivered by a good mother, while frustration of the child's wants and demands comes from a different, bad mother. Since the child cannot tolerate its own feelings of rage at mother, it performs the simple dyadic reversal of seeing the bad mother as a persecutor who maliciously inflicts the suffering the child is feeling. This defense is called projection, meaning that the child projects what it experiences as bad in itself into the external world, and thus fills the other in fantasy with its own bad stuff. Once it has done this, the child feels itself the victim of attack from the externalized enemy. Klein calls this the "paranoid position," referring to the infantile impulse to find the source of badness outside oneself.

When cognitive development permits the infant to see that there is only one mother, who is sometimes gratifying and sometimes frustrating, the child is supposed by Klein to shift to what she calls the "depressive position," in which he now recognizes that his paranoid attacks on the bad mother have injured the good mother. Now the child feels himself to be responsible for badness, and for causing the loss of his beloved good mother. As is easy to see, this shift is simply a re-reversal of the dyadic relation, so that now badness resides in the child, and it is mother who is the victim. When the child is able to tolerate this guilty feeling, he rises to the moral level of being motivated by the injury he perceives himself to have inflicted, in what Klein calls "reparation." Thus, unlike Richard III, who thought the world owed him reparations, the maturing child realizes that it is he who owes reparations to those whom he has unfairly wronged, at least in fantasy, while in the grip of the paranoid position.

The depressive position, out of which we may initiate genuine reparation, that is, a healing of the hurts of others rather than nursing our own grudges, is quite hard for even adults to hold onto. It requires that we accept those memories and experiences in our lives in which we have gone through unwanted loss or frustration and been powerless to do anything about it. Our normal urge is to defend ourselves against this humiliating passivity and inferiority to the forces arrayed against us. We develop all sorts of grandiose self-images, as well as paranoid blamings of external enemies, to avoid simply undergoing the dreaded experience of loss, shame, and powerlessness that is required if we are ever to mourn and then let go of the unattainable object of our desire, whatever it might be or have once been.

In therapy we give several things to our patients. First, through interpretations of their defenses as well as the impulses of which they are unaware, we enlighten them intellectually and equip them to deal cognitively with the habits of mind into which they have fallen. By our act of interpretation, too, we do something still more powerful, namely, instead of responding dyadically to the patient, we model for her or him the sort of objective, nonjudgmental self-reflective move that sidesteps dyadic yes-or-no relations in favor of more complex multi-perspectival understandings. We do not ignore our patients' vengeful rage when it is directed at us, but neither do we get angry back, or defend ourselves, or, on the other hand, act forgiving and acquiescent. Rather, we inquire into the meanings of the rage, and bring them to the patients' attention when they cannot do it for themselves, once we have learned after long listening from what fantasy they may arise.

Equally if not more important, we offer ourselves as objects upon which the patients stage their favored unconscious fantasy scenarios. We become, in their minds, as the therapy intensifies, the object of their wishes for revenge, and by allowing ourselves to do so, we demonstrate to the patient that we can withstand the impulses in them that have frightened them by seeming so dangerous that they had to be kept out of conscious awareness. We let them see not only that they actually have genuinely wished to kill one or another of their ambivalently beloved parents, for example, but also that they have not done so. By allowing them to express their wrath at us, and showing up alive for the next session, we let them experience the fact that their hidden revenge fantasy is not as lethal as they thought it was, and so to embark on the road from the paranoid to the depressive position.

Finally, by providing an atmosphere within which the patient feels able to go through what he or she had previously felt sure were intolerable experiences of loss, impotence, and humiliation in our presence, we allow the patient an opportunity to mourn loss, to feel and survive finitude, and to realize that there exist partial gradations between all and nothing where the rest of humanity lives.

They may not then give up entirely their fantasies of revenge, but their appreciation for the common lot, and especially for the human complexity in reality of even their most hated nemesis in fantasy, opens for them a psychic space within which inner psychological reconciliation is at least possible. The dominance of dyadic power struggles give way to more nuanced triadic relations or, as the Lacanians put it, the imaginary relation is superseded by the symbolic, for which the analyst has stood as placeholder and guarantor. We may never forgive, and our enemy may never apologize or feel our fury or confront our accusation; but we can forgive ourselves enough to enter into the circle of human social life without feeling we first have to redeem ourselves by a vengeful setting right of a long past shameful humiliation which, whatever its reality, is not so vital as to negate our future possibilities for full participation in our brief and difficult passage through this life.

Bibliography

Freud, Sigmund. "The Exceptions." In *The Standard Edition of the Complete Psychological Works of Sigmund Freud*, ed. J. Strachey. Vol. 14, pp. 311–315. London: Hogarth Press, 1966–74.

Klein, Melanie, and Joan Riviere. *Love, Hate and Reparation*. New York: Norton, 1964.

Segal, Hanna. *Introduction to the Work of Melanie Klein*. London: Karnac and the Institute of Psycho-Analysis, 1988.

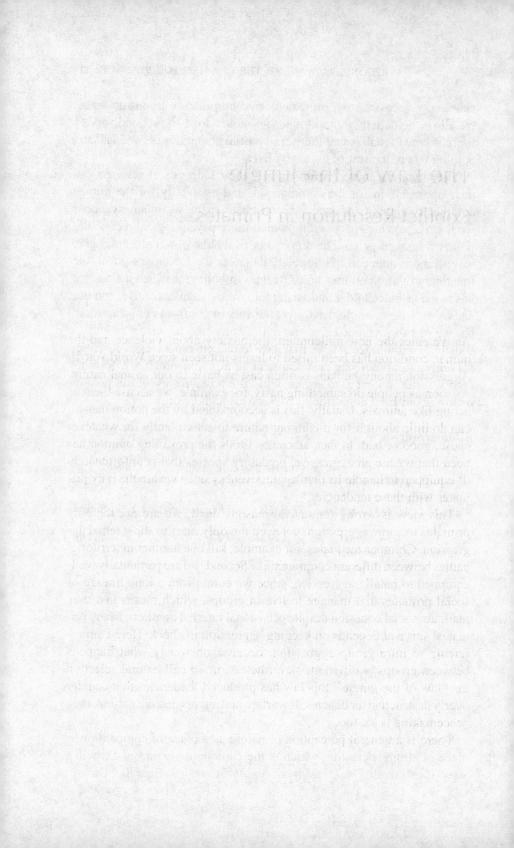

The Law of the Jungle

Conflict Resolution in Primates

Frans B.M. de Waal

As we enter the new millennium, the anxiety about violence and the human condition has been raised to levels not seen since World War II. Aggression among humans is often cast as basic to our animal nature. As soon as people do something nasty, for example, we accuse them of acting like animals. Usually, this is accompanied by the notion that we can do little about it for it is in our nature to act violently for whatever cause, good or bad. In fact, since the 1960s the prevailing opinion has been that we are an aggressive, predatory species that is unfortunately ill-equipped to handle its own aggressiveness since we are the only primates with these tendencies.[1]

This view is wrong for several reasons. First, we are not the only primates to show aggression, not even the only ones to show lethal aggression. Chimpanzee males, for example, kill one another in territorial battles between different communities.[2] Second, we are particularly well-equipped to handle aggression, since we come from a long lineage of social primates that manage to live in groups, which means that they maintain social cohesion despite occasional internal conflicts. Many primates' survival depends on keeping aggression in check. Here I am referring to intra-group aggression, because obviously what happens between groups is different. Nevertheless, if we call natural selection the "law of the jungle," this law has produced tendencies that counter overly destructive tendencies. If warfare and aggression are natural, then peacemaking is so, too.[3]

There is a general perception of nature as a place of competition, a place of struggle for life, which is the cardboard version of Darwin's view. If one reads *The Descent of Man*, however, it is clear that Darwin allowed for tendencies other than competitive ones. Darwin theorized that our morality also has evolutionary roots.[4] In the last two or three decades, however, many biologists have deviated from Darwin by presenting the natural world as a place of combat, a place where there is little room for anything that is nice or kind, and certainly not for reconciliation. This is a biased view that fortunately is not as dominant as it used to be. We are beginning to see the work of people who believe, like me, that in nature there is actually a lot of cooperation, with room for reconciliation, even morality.

Ecosystems

In nature, a lot of bargains are being struck between organisms. As a result we speak of ecosystems for a good reason. We do not speak of eco-collections; we call them ecosystems because everything is intertwined with everything else.

You are one of the many organisms who rely on other organisms for survival. Your whole intestinal system is relying on other organisms to do work for you. You have an entire flora and fauna inside of you. Also, our bodies are made up of cells, but cells may well be mergers of organelles that have gotten together and in which some types have come under the control of other ones.[5] Even at the cellular level, cooperation takes place and bargains are struck. Sometimes these bargains are exploitive rather than cooperative. For example, parasites are exploitive. While not all inter-organismal relationships are cooperative, many of them carry mutual benefits.

I should probably not be talking about ants in a volume in which Edward Wilson appears, but the ant world is a good place to see symbiosis at work. In Figure 1, we see ants and aphids; the ants protect the aphids, who have no weaponry and cannot defend themselves, and would therefore be easy food for all sorts of predators. In return, the aphids give the ants honeydew, so they act as a kind of cattle. Some ant species are completely dependent on them—they have aphid–milk cows that they milk for their honeydew. This sort of cooperation, in which there is mutual benefit, is very common in the insect world and at all sorts of levels. Another example is ants and acacias. The acacia bush is covered with ants, which live in and on it. In this co-evolved system, the acacia provides a sort of nectar at the base of its leaves to the ants, and provides thorns that are used as nests by the ants. The ants clean the acacia and

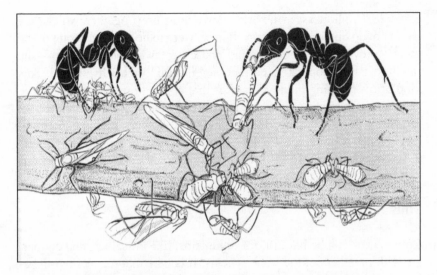

Figure 1. Symbiosis between different species is common in nature. Here, worker European wood ants attend aphids. (Drawing by Turid Forsyth in E.O. Wilson, *The Insect Societies* [Cambridge, MA: Harvard University Press, 1971]).

keep predators like caterpillars away. Scientists did experiments in the early part of the twentieth century in which they removed all the ants from acacias, and the bushes died. And the mutual benefits of the system extend beyond bush and ant: by eating the acacia beans, baboons help to disperse the seeds, and thus propagate the plants. Many plants are reliant on animals to some degree for seed dispersal, fertilization, and pollination. The number of collaborations going on to the mutual advantage of multiple organisms means that we cannot look at nature as just a place of competition. It is as much a place of cooperation.

Furthermore, competition can confer mutual benefits. We can look at competition in two ways. One is a win-lose situation, which is typical, for example, in territorial birds: one bird enters the territory and chases the other out or, more typically, is being chased back out by the territorial owner. In this kind of situation, one party wins, the other loses, and there is nothing in between. Although this situation occurs within human society sometimes, it is not the most common situation. What is more common in our kinds of societies, and those of other primates, are non-zero-sum situations: ones that result in one winner and one loser, but also an area of overlapping interest in which both will lose if they compete. This kind of situation is typical for cooperative animals—for example, two lionesses who bring down large prey together, which they could not do on their own. If one lioness were to be very intolerant of the other—prevent her from feeding, chase her away, or injure her—she might lose her cooperative partner, and in turn lose her livelihood. This kind of overlapping interest requires that competition be restrained.

In short, the natural world is not purely a battlefield—the view promoted by Thomas Henry Huxley[6] and his followers among contemporary science popularizers. It also is a place of mutual dependency among different species as well as members of the same species. This means that conflict needs to be constrained.

Mutualism

Competition can be harmful for organisms, like ourselves, that cooperate with members of the same species. It is here that reconciliation becomes crucial: when there are both conflicting and overlapping interests. We can look at two forms of cooperation, mutualism and reciprocity, to gain a better understanding of the ways in which reconciliation and conflict resolution operate as the law of the jungle.

Mutualism is defined as a situation in which two parties perform actions toward the same goal and enjoy benefits at the same time. Being a very simple arrangement, mutualism is widespread in the animal kingdom. For example, pelicans are very cooperative animals that exercise a wonderful system of mutualism, as illustrated in Figure 2, a photograph from Kenya. In this photograph, all the white dots are birds, pelicans and flamingos. You can see pelicans swimming in a very well arranged semi-circle. The lake is very shallow and full of fish. The pelicans paddle their feet, which brings the fish together at the center of their semi-circle. Then they scoop them up and eat them together. If a pelican were to try to fish this way on its own, it would not get anywhere. And the system is simple—they all enjoy the benefits at the same time, so they do not need to keep track of who owes whom a favor. This sort of mutualistic arrangement is so common that we almost take it for granted—some of my colleagues start yawning when people talk about mutualism because they have heard so many examples of it. But while it is a very common arrangement, it is one that highlights the need to resolve conflicts: if these animals could not work together, they would have a much more difficult time. Put in this perspective, we see that sometimes survival depends on being able to work together.

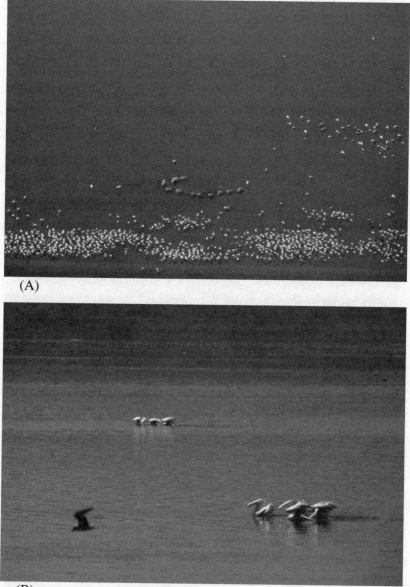

(A)

(B)

Figure 2 (a and b). White pelicans in a shallow lake, in Kenya, where these birds perform mutualistic cooperation. They form semicircles to capture fish driven together by the paddling birds' feet. Photograph A shows one such semi-circle. As soon as enough fish are concentrated in the center of the circle, the pelicans simultaneously scoop up the prey, shown on the right-hand side in Photograph B. (Photographs by the author.)

I now turn to an organism that is quite a bit smarter than pelicans and quite a bit closer to us: the chimpanzee. The chimpanzee is genetically almost identical to us. It has a very similar brain (although smaller than ours). When we look at chimpanzee society, we find that it alternates between competition and cooperation—even more than in many other species. Chimpanzee society is very intensive and dynamic, and it is in that sort of context that reconciliation takes place.

There are all sorts of rituals in place in the animal kingdom so that animals who could kill each other do not in fact do so. For example, there are poisonous snakes who fight with each other but do not use their fangs. In the same way, a male chimpanzee will not usually use his teeth when fighting with a female chimpanzee; he will, however, use his teeth if he is fighting with another male. There are all sorts of inhibitions and fighting rituals that form the first barrier against detrimental aggression.

Peacemaking

Another barrier against this kind of aggression is to repair and maintain relationships. Figure 3 shows what happens after a fight—in this case between two male chimpanzees who have been screaming at each other. About ten minutes after the fight, one of them holds out a hand, inviting the other one for contact. About a second later, they embrace and kiss each other—that is the reconciliation. Apes and monkeys do this differently. While monkeys make no eye contact with their opponent when they reconcile, humans and apes cannot reconcile without eye contact. If you were to have a fight with a colleague, and you were reconciling with that person but he or she would not look at you—looking instead at the ceiling or the floor or somewhere else—you would not feel reconciled with that partner. You would feel that there is still something wrong. Thus, eye contact as a test of feelings and intentions is a critical part of the process. In chimpanzees this often proceeds to a mouth-to-mouth kiss, which is the typical way they reconcile.

It is not hard to understand why reconciliation was discovered in chimpanzees: the pattern is very human-like, and so we recognize it easily. But we have data on more than twenty-five different primate species in which reconciliation occurs—not just in apes but also in many monkey species. The same sort of studies have been done with human children, and of course they show these kinds of behaviors also—not necessarily in this particular way, but they do have ways of reconciling. Some re-

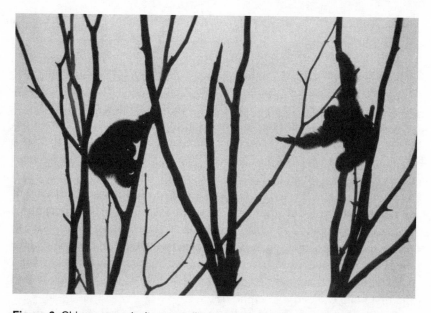

Figure 3. Chimpanzees invite reconciliation by means of eye contact and hand gestures. This photograph shows the situation ten minutes after a protracted, noisy conflict between two adult males at the Arnhem Zoo. The challenged male (left) fled into a tree. He is now being approached by his opponent, who stretches out a hand. Within seconds, the two males have a physical reunion and climb down together to groom each other on the ground. (Photograph by the author.)

searchers have even found reconciliation in dolphins, hyenas, and some other nonprimates. I recently received a letter from someone who is preparing to study reconciliation practices in salamanders. This means that in cooperative species, reconciliation may be very widespread and not limited to primates—possibly not even limited to mammals. It may be a fairly common mechanism that exists where relationships need to be maintained despite occasional conflict.[7]

The definition of reconciliation that we use in this kind of research is a friendly reunion between former opponents not long after a conflict. This differs somewhat from the general definition of social reconciliation among humans, primarily because we look for a definition that we can measure in observational studies. In our case, the stipulation is that the reunion happen not long after the conflict. There is no intrinsic reason that reconciliation could not occur after hours or days, or, in the case of humans, even after generations. We have seen that sort of reconciliation: The pope has gone places to reconcile fifty years, or even more than a millennium, after the initial problem. In theory, nonhuman primates might also reconcile years after the event of conflict, but that is a difficult proposal to study.

Before I go into some experimental studies, let me first illustrate a few aspects of reconciliation. So far as I know, chimpanzees are the only animals who use mediators in conflict resolution. In order to be able to mediate conflict, you have to understand relationships outside of yourself; that may be the reason that other animals fail to show this aspect of conflict resolution. For example, if two male chimpanzees have been involved in a fight, even on a very large island as where I did my studies, they cannot easily avoid each other, but instead sit opposite from each other and avoid eye contact. They can sit like this for a long time. (I think this is the sort of situation that President Jimmy Carter often deals with between countries in conflict—a standoff in which neither party wants to take the first step to reconcile.) In this situation, it is the females who move in and try to solve the issue. A female moves over to one of the males and grooms him for a brief while. She then gets up and walks very slowly to the other male, and the first male walks right behind her.

We have seen situations in which, if the first male failed to follow, the female turned around to grab his arm and make him follow. So the process of getting the two males in proximity seems intentional on the part of the female. She then begins grooming the other male, and the first male grooms her, so there are three chimpanzees grooming each other. Before long, she disappears from the scene and the males continue grooming: she has in effect brought the two parties together.

This kind of conflict mediation was observed about twenty-five times at the zoo where I worked, and at the Yerkes Primate Center we have recently seen cases as well. It is always the same configuration in terms of gender: adult males are in conflict and the mediator is a female. This kind of transaction requires that the female understand what happened between the males, that there is an issue that can be resolved, and that she be able to resolve it. It requires a lot of social awareness and diplomacy and authority—usually older females do this, not young ones. And it reveals the level of sophistication and understanding that is involved in conflict resolution in a chimpanzee society.

Valuable Relationships

The central hypothesis that we have worked with in the field of conflict resolution in animals—and I would argue that the same hypothesis applies equally to humans—is that reconciliation will occur especially between parties who stand much to lose if their relationship deteriorates. Reconciliation is not done because you want to be nice or to be happy together; it is done for very practical reasons. If you do not repair the relationship, you both have much to lose. This non-zero-sum principle is widely used in the study of animals, and is familiar to people as well. I would propose that even the European Union (EU) is based on this principle. The EU was formed after much warfare in Europe. Some visionary politicians then argued that fostering economic ties between the nations may prevent warfare because there will be too much at stake, too much to lose if, say, Germany invaded France, or vice versa. When your economy's success is linked to that of another people, you have a reason not to go to war with them. I would argue that this principle, which we think applies within primate societies, applies in all sorts of systems.

Here are a few data points that support this position. The first one is a study on macaques. Macaques are primates that practice reconciliation, but some species within the genus practice it more than others. The best known macaque, the rhesus monkey, is not known for being a particularly conciliatory species (Figure 4). Marina Cords has recently done an interesting experiment with a species that is very similar in temperament, the longtailed macaque, in which she manipulated the value of relationships among monkeys. She brought pairs of monkeys into a cage, provided them with a popcorn machine, and arranged it so that they could only eat from the popcorn machine if they came together. As a result, she trained these monkeys to become cooperative. Because they had to depend on having a partner to get food, they placed a higher value on relationships. She did a follow-up experiment in which she would induce competition between them—by throwing food to them—and then measure the conciliatory tendencies after the fight. She had a control group in which the monkeys lived in the same circumstances but could feed from the machine independently. The investigators found a sharply increased tendency to reconcile after fights in the noncontrol group. They found in this experiment that if you make the relationship more valuable between parties, you will increase the peacemaking tendencies.[8]

We also have evidence that reconciliation is not purely an instinct, that it is instead a social skill that can be acquired—and thus can be instilled or removed based on culture or environment. I performed an

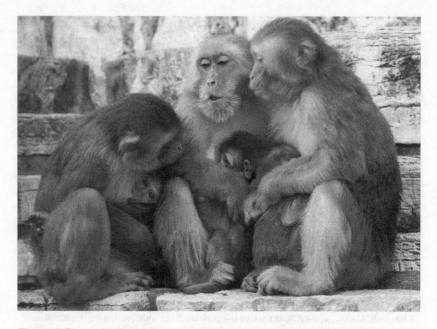

Figure 4. Reconciliations allow rhesus monkeys to maintain tight kinship bonds despite frequent intrafamilial squabbles. Shortly after two adult sisters bit each other, they reunite sitting on the left and right of their mother, the alpha female of the troop, each female holding her own infant. The sisters lipsmack while the matriarch loudly grunts. (Photograph by the author.)

experiment on this idea of flexibility of character using eight young rhesus monkeys and stumptail monkeys. Rhesus monkeys reconcile after fights to some degree, but they are not nearly as conciliatory as stumptail monkeys. We housed these two species together for five months. If you put monkeys of these species together, at first you get a sort of segregated society in which the rhesus sleep in one corner and the stumptails in another, and never the two will meet. In fact, they are afraid of each other. By the end of five months, however, if they are together day and night, a fully integrated group emerges. They sleep together, play together, and groom together. After five months, we set about separating them again, and then measuring the effect of that time together on conciliatory behavior.

Our results are shown in Figure 5. First, in the research controls—rhesus monkeys who are just living with each other—there was no change in the tendency to reconcile during the whole period of the experiment. The tendency remained relatively low, as expected. From other experi-

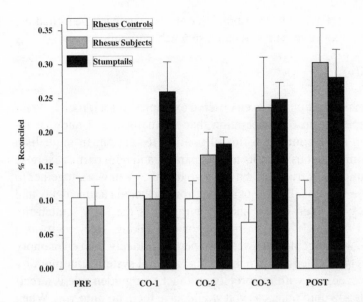

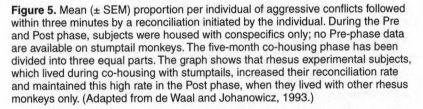

Figure 5. Mean (± SEM) proportion per individual of aggressive conflicts followed within three minutes by a reconciliation initiated by the individual. During the Pre and Post phase, subjects were housed with conspecifics only; no Pre-phase data are available on stumptail monkeys. The five-month co-housing phase has been divided into three equal parts. The graph shows that rhesus experimental subjects, which lived during co-housing with stumptails, increased their reconciliation rate and maintained this high rate in the Post phase, when they lived with other rhesus monkeys only. (Adapted from de Waal and Johanowicz, 1993.)

ments, we know that stumptails on their own have a high rate of reconciliation. The experimental rhesus monkeys—those living with the stumptails—start out at the same low level as the rhesus controls. In the first period of co-housing, they have the same level of reconciliatory behavior. But after they have lived with the stumptails, and after we have segregated them again so that they are living only with rhesus monkeys who went through the same experience, we see that these rhesus reconcile as much as the stumptails do. So, we have created a "new and improved" rhesus monkey, one that reconciles much more easily than the regular rhesus monkey.[9]

This is in effect an experiment with social culture: We have changed the social culture of a group of rhesus monkeys and made it more similar to that of stumptail monkeys by exposing the former to the practices of this other species. This experiment also shows that there exists great flexibility in behavior; it gives hope that if you can teach peacemaking to rhesus monkeys, maybe you can also teach it to children.

Reciprocity

In the animal kingdom, we even observe examples of reciprocity—a far more complex form of cooperation than mutualism, and one that requires even more complex forms of conflict resolution. In mutualism there are simultaneous benefits to both parties, and both parties exercise a certain amount of trust in each other so that they can work together to obtain these benefits. But in social reciprocity, there is a time delay and contingency between giving and receiving. It is the "you scratch my back and I'll scratch yours" principle of turn-taking. Reciprocity is a transactional arrangement between two parties who rely both on memory and on an enforcement system that is also a moral system. Our morality is very preoccupied with reciprocity—in fact, our golden rule is a reciprocity rule: do unto others as you would have them do unto you. When we use the word "obligation," we use a moral term related to reciprocity. We have moral systems to reinforce reciprocity, an issue now increasingly studied in animals.

In a recent study of reciprocity that I conducted, we examined capuchin monkeys. These monkeys are very small, hence easy to work with, but nevertheless have large brains. They are so smart and manipulative that they are sometimes called the South American chimpanzee. We know that they hunt cooperatively, like chimpanzees do, so we decided to look at reciprocity by mimicking cooperative hunts—not by giving them an animal to hunt, but by providing them with a situation in which they could cooperate and in which only one individual obtains the rewards, as typical of group hunts.

The experiment required the monkeys to do what, for capuchins, is a simple task: we took two of them out of the group they lived in, put them in a test chamber divided into two sections by a mesh panel, and provided them with a tray that they could pull in. We made the tray so heavy that one monkey could not pull it in alone. Then we put food in cups on the tray—one cup for each side of the mesh panel. If you put food in both cups, this becomes a mutualism experiment in which both parties enjoy benefits at the same time. The capuchins in the experiment did that very easily: everyone wanted to pull to get food. But then we took away one cup and made the experiment more interesting. If there is food only in one cup, then both monkeys are pulling, but only one monkey is rewarded. They engage in this kind of cooperation much less frequently, but they engage in it nonetheless.

We found that after they had pulled the food in to the one monkey, that monkey would share his food with his pulling-partner through the mesh. We then measured how much the monkey who got the food was willing to share with the partner who helped him or her get it, and with that measure we were able to understand something about reciprocity.

In our experiment we measured the differences in sharing between two situations: the one just described and a control experiment, in which the second partner's help is not needed (dubbed "solo pulls"). Every session had four trials. In the first trial, the monkeys who participated in cooperative efforts shared more food than the control group, in which only one monkey had a pull bar and only one monkey needed to pull. There was much less sharing there. The same was true for the later trials. We dubbed this effect payment for labor: the monkey who needed and received assistance was more willing to share with the partner than when the partner was not needed.[10]

Such experiments seem to reveal a system of reciprocity in which there may be an understanding of what a service means and that that service needs to be rewarded if it is to happen again. In animals with sophisticated social systems, you see systems of reciprocity rather than mutualism; and these systems of reciprocity require forms of conflict resolution that are quite a bit more sophisticated. There is even more need for reconciliation—and more need for keeping tabs on partners, knowing what have they done for the other partner lately—in these situations. Reconciliation is then a strategic move in which the benefits of the relationship figure heavily. Conversely, if there are no benefits in the relationship, reconciliation may be undesirable.

So, despite the fact that conflicting interests can sometimes create tension, reconciliation serves to maintain cooperation and mutual benefits despite these tensions. Reconciliation allows the continuation of cooperation between parties with occasionally clashing interests. But perhaps this idea is more interesting when we turn it around: conflicts of interest among mutually dependent parties can be expressed, negotiated, and settled thanks to mechanisms of conflict resolution. In other words, we have societies in which we value competition within our economic systems. We have democracies because we realize that not everyone has the same opinion and we need to test and sample opinions before we decide on things. So we have designed social systems that acknowledge competition and conflicts of interest between parties. And we can only form these social systems because we have mechanisms like reconciliation and compromise. If we did not have those mechanisms in place, we would not be able to form the sorts of societies that we have; our relationships would be completely chaotic—there would be no way of overcoming all the conflicts of interest that exist to reach the goals of the society.

While the previous essay in this volume explored the ancient roots of the revenge impulse, the message I wish to impart is that compromise, reconciliation skills, and conflict resolution skills are also very old. They have deep biological roots in the sense that they go back millions of years. Reconciliation is not something that we came up with because of some novel intelligence, or thanks to religion, or because we can look further into the future than animals. It is a category of behavior that arose long before we appeared on this planet. We may have reached levels that are perhaps more advanced than in a chimpanzee or any other animal, but we are making use of an old psychology.

Notes

1. See R.A. Ardrey, *The Territorial Imperative* (London, Collins, 1967). Also, Ardrey, "The Violent Way," *Life*, September 11, 1970, 56–68; and K.Z. Lorenz, *On Aggression* (London: Methuen, 1963 [reprint]).

2. R.W. Wrangham and D. Peterson, *Demonic Males: Apes and the Evolution of Human Aggression* (Boston: Houghton Mifflin, 1996).

3. F.B.M. de Waal, *Peacemaking Among Primates* (Cambridge, MA: Harvard University Press, 1989).

4. C. Darwin, *The Descent of Man, and Selection in Relation to Sex* (Princeton, NJ: Princeton University Press, 1981 [1871]).

5. L. Margulis, *Symbiotic Planet: A New Look at Evolution* (New York: Basic Books, 1998).

6. T.H. Huxley, *Evolution and Ethics* (Princeton, NJ: Princeton University Press, 1989 [1894]).

7. F. Aureli and F.B.M. de Waal, *Natural Conflict Resolution* (Berkeley: University of California Press, 2000). See also F.B.M. de Waal, "Primates—A Natural Heritage of Conflict Resolution," *Science* 289 (2000): 586–590.

8. M. Cords and S. Thurnheer, "Reconciling with Valuable Partners by Long-Tailed Macaques," *Ethology* 93 (1993): 315–325.

9. F.B.M. de Waal and D.L. Johanowicz, "Modification of Reconciliation Behavior Through Social Experience: An Experiment with Two Macaque Species," *Child Development* 64 (1993): 897–908.

10. F.B.M. de Waal and M.L. Berger, "Payment for Labour in Monkeys," *Nature* 404 (2000): 563.

Reflections on the Future of Life

E.O. Wilson

My subject in this essay is the type of reconciliation that is closest to my heart: reconciliation between humanity and nature, between our species and the rest of the world. Have you ever wondered how we will be remembered a thousand years from now, when we seem as remote as Charlemagne? Most, I believe, would choose something like the following: techno-scientific revolution; ongoing, globalized, unstoppable; computer capacity approaching that of the human brain, expected to match it in twenty to thirty years; semi-autonomous robots at work; genetic engineering perfected; space colonized; overpopulation slackening; governments turning to democracy; trade globalized; people better fed and healthier.

In this buoyant view of the early twenty-first century, what might we have overlooked about our place in history? What might we be neglecting and at risk of losing forever? In the year 3000, I believe the most likely answer will be: much of the rest of life—of the creation, if you prefer; a lot of our environmental security; and, just as important, part of what it means to be human. In just the past twenty to thirty years, scientists have found the biosphere to be richer in diversity than ever before conceived. Biodiversity, which took over 3 billion years to evolve, is being eroded at an accelerating rate by human activity. In any encapsulated summary of how we will be remembered, that loss will inflict a heavy price in wealth, security, and spirit.

The bottom line in global economics differs from that generally assumed by our leading economists and philosophers; they have mostly ignored the numbers that count. While the United Nations estimates that our world population of more than 6 billion will peak at 8–10 billion by mid-century (before it starts to descend), the amount of per capita fresh water and arable land are dropping to levels that resource experts agree are very risky.[1]

The key statistic is the ecological footprint, which is the average amount of productive land in coastal marine environment appropriated by each person, but not in a single block. This includes land around where you live, say in Massachusetts or Georgia, but also bits and pieces from around the world needed to produce your food, water, housing, energy and transport, commerce, and waste management. Each person, for example, draws on a little bit of land in Costa Rica for coffee, a little bit of Saudi Arabia for oil, and so on. The ecological footprint of the average person in the developing world, which includes more about 5 billion of the earth's 6 billion people, is about two and a half acres. The ecological footprint of the average person in the United States is ten times as much, about twenty-four acres.[2] With our present levels of technology, if every person in the world were to reach American levels of consumption, we would need to have four more planet earths. I stress this fact because there is still the notion floating around in the discussion of our consumption that the human biomass is extremely small and that we have more than enough space left on the ice-free surface of the earth.

The people of developing countries may never want to attain our level of profligacy, but in simply trying to achieve a decent standard of living, they have joined the industrial world in converting the last of the natural environments and reducing a large part of the planet's fauna and flora to endangered status or into final extinction. At the same time, Homo sapiens has become a geophysical force, the first species ever to do that. We have driven atmospheric carbon dioxide to the highest level in at least 200,000 years. We have unbalanced the nitrogen cycle, have thinned the protective ozone layer of the atmosphere, and have triggered—without any reasonable doubt—global warming that will ultimately be bad news everywhere. Our destruction of the natural environment began a long time ago in what can be described as a mistaken capital investment. Having appropriated the earth's natural resources during the Neolithic revolution (starting around 10,000 years ago), humanity chose to annuitize the resources with a progressively increasing payoff. We have gulped down our capital faster and faster, like a wastrel heir to an unearned fortune.

At the time it seemed a wise decision; viewed in the short term, as on the pages of the *Wall Street Journal*, it still does. After all, the result is rising per capita production and consumption—markets awash in oil and grain. And optimistic economists are monitoring the GDPs and comparative indexes for us. But there is a problem.

The key elements of natural capital—that is, everything that underlies the market economy, including earth's arable land, our ground water, forests, marine fisheries, petroleum, and so forth—are finite. And they are not subject to proportionate capital growth. They are furthermore being decapitalized by overharvesting, habitat destruction, and soil erosion. Therefore, with population and consumption continuing to increase, the per capita amounts of resources left to be harvested are falling and destined to do so at an increasingly faster pace in the future. The long-term prospects are not promising. This is the answer to the oft-repeated response to environmentalists that in spite of all their dire predictions, things are still getting better and better.

Humanity, which has at last awakened to the realities of the natural economy, the foundation of our capital economy, has begun an earnest search for alternative sources of materials and energies. In the final analysis, I think the twenty-first century will be the century of the environment. It will be the time when we must put our house in order and settle down before we wreck the planet. The immediate future is usefully conceived as a bottleneck. Science and technology, combined with a lack of self-understanding and a paleolithic obstinacy that have led to ruinous environmental practices, have brought us to where we are today. Now, science and technology, combined with foresight and moral courage—both based upon a more enlightened ethic—must see us through the bottleneck and out of it. One hopes this will happen by the end of the century.

There are two collateral effects for the bottleneck phenomenon worth keeping in mind, and congruent to the subject of reconciliation. The first is that the rich grow richer and the poor grow poorer. The income difference between the one-fifth of the world's population in the wealthiest countries and the one-fifth of the population in the poorest countries was 30:1 in 1960, 60:1 in 1990, and 74:1 in the year 2000.[3] Eight hundred million people remain in what the United Nations classifies as absolute poverty—no sanitation, no clean water, rampant disease, periodic starvation, child mortality in the tens of thousands per week. The income differential is often dismissed as a humanitarian issue, but it should be considered a security issue: it is a setting for resentment and fanaticism, and the arrival of heaven-bent suicide bombers.

The second collateral effect—the one to which I have paid a lot of attention in my work—is the acceleration of the natural environment in leading to the mass extinction of ecosystems and species. The damage already done cannot be repaired within any period of time that has meaning for the human mind. The more it is allowed to grow, the more future generations will suffer for it in ways both well understood now and still unimagined. The radical reduction of the world's biodiversity is the folly for which our descendents are the least likely to forgive us.

What Is Biodiversity? How Much of It Is There?

Let me review some of the basic facts concerning biological diversity, or biodiversity for short. First of all, I define biodiversity as simply the expression for all the forms of life examined at the different levels of biological organization. How much biodiversity is there? If you just consider the Australian ecosystem, from rain forests to mangroves, to shallow marine areas and all the species that occupy it, there are somewhere between 1.5 and 1.8 million species. And this includes only species we know well enough to have given scientific names and for which we have determined at least a rudimentary anatomical diagnosis. This number is not exact because a full census has not been attempted, and we can only note generalities in the kinds of organisms that make up the bulk of biodiversity, especially insects. The main photosynthetic organisms in diversity are, as you would expect, the flowering plants. But we should note that this is due in large part to the intricate and complex co-evolution within those groups that has occurred since the end of the Mesozoic era, about 70–90 million years ago in geologic time.

Another way to begin to grasp biodiversity is to consider the size of organisms relative to their population in the world. And so the beetle, representing insects, looms like a Goodyear blimp above the tiny elephant, which represents our 5,000 known mammal species. The elephant hides beneath a tree-sized fungus, which is even an understatement: 60,000 species of known fungi are really only a small fraction of the estimated 1.6 million species of fungi that exist. The point of this is that we do not know, to the nearest order of magnitude, the number of species, of organisms that live on earth. This might be as low as 5 or 6 million, but that is highly unlikely; it might be as high as 100 million, or even higher as we get to know microbial biodiversity even better.[4] Some say that a good figure to settle on is

10 million, but no biologist knows with any degree of confidence if that is a good number.

Another exercise in perspective helps here: If you were to take out the four strands of DNA of a typical body cell and put them in real space, you would have a single molecule about a meter long, which you could not see because it would be 2 billionths of a meter across. If you magically magnified that DNA from a human cell until it was the width of a piece of string, it would extend approximately 1,800 miles, the distance from New York to Dallas. As you walk along, you would be reading off the genetic letters, the nucleotide pairs, at about 100 per inch. That is the information in an organism; it is something to bear in mind when we allow a species to go extinct.

Thanks to breakthroughs in genomics and exponentially increasing technical power, we can now perform a full gene inventory of species. We are on the edge of being able to go out and study bacteria in the field, in the woods, on the street, in front of this building, where you would expect to find hundreds of thousands of species. Quite soon, it will be possible to pick up that pinch of soil and, in a relatively short period of time—a few days, maybe a week or two—read the thousands of species that are in it. Because of these advances in identifying organisms, we are about to make a breakthrough in our understanding of biodiversity.

Where Is Biodiversity Located?

The ecology rule tells us that biodiversity occurs wherever there is liquid water or even the potential of liquid water. This means that there is biodiversity from pole to pole, from the summit of Everest to the lowest depths of 35,000 feet beneath the ocean's surface. At the very least there exists bacteria and other micro-organisms there, some of which also thrive in water above the boiling point. In fact, there is one species living in thermal vents on the sea floor that ceases reproducing when you *lower* the temperature of water to the boiling point. There are microscopic creatures thriving two miles or more below the surface of the water, drawing energy from the metabolism of inorganic chemicals.[5] This means that even if everything were eliminated from the surface of the earth, if it became a blasted, seared cinder, there would still be organisms below living on.

Most of the species of known organisms occur in the tropical rain forests, ecosystems that cover only about 6 percent of the earth's land surface; this is down to about half of the area of rain forests that existed before humanity started cutting them. As an ecosystem, the rain forest is a fabulous treasury of species of plants, animals, and microorganisms that are just beginning to be explored. Much of that is concentrated in the canopy, an area that has only recently been reached effectively by biologists because it is so difficult to get to. Many of the trees that dominate the rain forest have smooth trunks or trunks with lots of spines on them, and they go straight up for seventy feet or more before they branch. And once you get up there, you run into the epiphyte gardens, where orchids or even cacti grow. The young, athletic scientists making this area their specialty have to be able to get up there first, then push their way through spiny and nettle-like leaves amid swarms of stinging wasps and ants. Tarzan would not have lasted fifteen minutes as a rain forest biologist.[6] But these young scientists, who are of course thrilled to be there, work along the edge of the canopy, high above the ground where most of the photosynthesis takes place and forms of life exist that have never been seen before. This is a true physical frontier of science.

It is here in the rain forests that we are doing the most damage to the diversity of life, easily illustrated in the clear-cutting of the Brazilian rain forest, which has resulted in the mass destruction of habitats for species we have not yet even discovered. I like to use the mnemonic device of the acronym HIPPO to describe the damage: The H stands for the most damaging kind of destruction—habitat destruction. The I stands for "introduction of alien species," which I discuss further below. The Ps stand for pollution and population (really overpopulation), a root cause that exacerbates these other problems. And the O stands for overharvesting.

The rain forests of the state of São Paulo in Brazil offer an unfortunately typical story of habitat destruction. This great forest, because it lies along the Atlantic coast of Brazil, is distinct from the Amazonian forest—it has quite different plants, animals, and so on. When Darwin visited there in 1832, he was thrilled by the beauty and majesty of this forest. But with the settlement of the Atlantic coast, it was aggressively cut; today, there is less than 10 percent of the original forest left. Brazilians are now engaged in an emergency rescue, stabilizing the forest of their beloved—and now much better appreciated—*mata atlantica*.

Another example is found in the rain forests of the Philippines. The destruction of these ecosystems is ongoing. The forest cover shrank over the last century—to 10 percent of its original cover—and this continues. Whole islands have been denuded; as a result, plants and animals that were unique to the Philippine Islands—their natural heritage—are disappearing swiftly. I dwell on the subject of the rain forest because we believe that more than half the species on earth live there; this habitat must be taken as a prototype, a paradigm for what can happen when habitats are threatened. The tropical rain forests are disappearing worldwide at the rate of 0.5 to 1 percent a year. The remaining area that the rain forests all over the world cover is about equal to the contiguous 48 states; the rate of destruction is equal to about half or all of the state of Florida every year. This translates to as much as a quarter of 1 percent of species extinguished or committed to extinction each year (meaning that there are a few individuals still found but they will soon disappear).

So we see, without doubt, that we have been destroying habitats at an ever increasing pace all over the world. But what is the exact consequence of this destruction of habitat? We can see the answer in the principle worked out by ecologists in what they have called the area-species curves. Reptiles and amphibians found on the different islands of the West Indies offer one example. As we go from the very large islands of Cuba and Hispaniola to middle-size islands like Jamaica and Puerto Rico, right down to the very small islands of the Lesser Antilles, we find that as the area is reduced, the number of species that exist also shrinks. In general, when the amount of reduction of the habitat area reaches 90 percent, there is a reduction of half of the species.[7]

This principle also holds true for habitat islands—places that are not necessarily land surrounded by sea, but are habitats unique to a particular area. What is true on islands in a sea holds true on mountaintops surrounded by coniferous forest, or a lake surrounded by land. This is particularly bad news for the national parks systems all over the world; we learn that we cannot assume that once we set aside an area to be protected from development and destruction, we have kept biodiversity safe for all time. The national parks of the western United States and southwestern Canada are habitat islands, natural environment surrounded by seas of the developed, disturbed land of ranches and farms. During the last 100 years, the record shows that overall, the species of mammals found in these parks have been declining.[8] Just as the theoreticians predicted, those in the large islands are declining less rapidly, and those in the smallest islands are declining quite rapidly. Eventually, we expect that they will come out to a new equilibrium. But we are losing species even in our most protected reserves.

So it turns out that clear-cutting is not the only way to damage what could otherwise be a protected area. Damage also occurs when you cut *into* a forest—for example, to put roads through it, which is happening more frequently in the greatest of all the tropical forest wildernesses, the Amazon-Orinoco Basin. If a forest is cut with a semi-natural area left around it, it may be able to recover by growing back slowly from the edge. But if it is cut sharply, we get what is called the edge effect, a drying out of as much as a kilometer from the edge, and the dying off of trees that are adapted to deep forests and the creatures that live with them. What happens when these trees are left at the edge of a forest is that they are damaged—by winds that come up and blow down trees or decapitate the canopy, and by species of weeds that choke them out. So if we cut the forest incorrectly, we find that it retreats spontaneously thereafter.

Reckoning the Damage

We are just beginning to understand the impact of alien species on habitats: that they are truly destructive to the environment at an increasing rate. Sometimes deliberately and sometimes inadvertently, we have begun to homogenize the fauna and flora of the world by introducing alien species that push back native species and change the environment. One important example of such an alien species is the fire ant, brought from South America to the American South, and now altering the environment from the Carolinas to Texas, pushing native species back. On a personal note, in 1942, when I was thirteen years old, I made my first published scientific finding: I identified colonies of imported red fire ants. I was doing a survey of the ants in my neighborhood, and I found these ants and became familiar with them. Six years later I was hired as a student at the University of Alabama by the state of Alabama's Department of Conservation to do a survey. It became clear to me that in 1942 these ants had probably been around just for a few years and they might have been limited to that one area. (If I had done my duty, I would have put on a pair of long pants and told somebody, "You know, if you wipe out these ants now, you are going to save millions of dollars in the future." But that never occurred to me.)

We can also cite examples from a long list of the most destructive, invasive species—a list that one ecologist calls America's Least Wanted. One animal would be the brown tree snake, which wiped out all of the native songbirds of Guam after it was introduced from New Guinea some fifty years ago. Another is Miconia, which is also called the green cancer; it is a native of the American tropics that has crowded out almost all plants and animals in many habitats of parts of French Polynesia.

We can use three separate measures to figure out how fast species are becoming extinct. First is the area-species curve I have described. Another method uses the status of individual species in the records kept by the International Union for Conservation of Nature. These species descend on a trajectory of categories from vulnerable to endangered to critically endangered and then to extinct. We can track how quickly they descend from one category to the next. The third method is to make a prognosis based on the current condition of endangered species in the population analysis. It has been estimated that the current rate of extinction is between 100 and 10,000 times higher than it was before the coming of humanity.[9] Some believe—and I am among them—that even these numbers are too low, the increase could be on the order of 10,000 or higher because as entire ecosystems are eliminated, their populations spiral down to zero. We have seen this happen in the rain forest on the Philippine island of Sabu, and we are seeing it happen more and more around the world. It is entirely possible, and some analysts even say likely, that if the present rates of habitat destruction and spread of alien species continue, we could lose half the species of plants and animals on earth by the end of the century.

What Can We Do?

At this moment in history we are challenged by the project of raising the lives of people everywhere to a decent level while preserving intact as much of the natural environment as possible. Most people see these two concerns—raising standards of living and preserving the natural world—as antithetical, as competing interests. But I would argue that the two goals are intertwined. They can be approached in a synergistic way in which progress in one enhances progress in the other.

I close this essay with some information from a dispatch from the Global Conservation Front that addresses the attempt to stop the hemorrhaging of ecosystems and species. First, it turns out that large blocks of the last remaining natural environment in wilderness areas can be preserved at surprisingly low cost and in such a way as to yield greater profit to the people and the countries owning them. These wilderness areas include the Amazon, the Congo, and New Guinea. Logging companies in these and other regions are operating on a very thin profit margin. They can be outbid by conservation groups using private gifts, which are then leveraged by grants from other nongovernmental organizations (NGOs) such as the Global Environmental Fund and the World Bank. And it won't take much to outbid the logging companies. For as little as $10 an acre (and often much less), conservation concessions can be established in which countries otherwise prepared to make logging concessions turn to preserve the forest instead. Or a trust fund can be set up with the proceeds being paid to the country for preserving and managing large reserves. Or the logging rights can be purchased in some places for as little as $2–3 an acre. But the environment is not the only benefactor: a good percentage of the local people in sparsely inhabited areas can be engaged in caring for the park, managing and guarding it. A typical salary for them might be as little as $100 a month. One of my colleagues who recently returned from the Dominican Republic has reported to me that people in the rural areas there consider a salary of $150 a month as really excellent. Finally, the land could be purchased outright.

By these means, two organizations alone—Conservation International and the Nature Conservancy—managed to add more than 2 million acres to the parks and reserves of Bolivia, Guyana, and Suriname. These groups are also offering research and management expertise to promote the use of this land, to help the residents yield greater income from tourism, carbon credits under the Kyoto agreements, and other noninvasive income sources that would be more profitable than timber leases and agricultural conversion. Other developing countries around the world are now exploring similar arrangements. It looks very promising.

Another point of entry is the preservation of hotspots, those particular forests, coral reefs, and other local habitats that both are endangered and contain the largest number of kinds of plants and animals found nowhere else. Just twenty-five of the terrestrial hotspots cover only 1.4 percent of the land surface of earth, but they are the exclusive home of an astonishing 44 percent of all known species of vascular plants and 36 percent of mammals, birds, reptiles, and amphibians. This "hotspot preservation" is the approach favored by Conservation International and the

World Wildlife Fund, among other American-based NGOs, to increase the effectiveness of conservation efforts in fund-raising and local economic and conservation management. There are going to be parts of the world, in these hotspots, that are not going to be so easily improved with raising the income of the people around them, however; one of them is in southern California.

It has become clear that progress in conservation everywhere, particularly global conservation, is dependent on joint enterprises of the private sector, government, and science. We have to know exactly what is at stake. We must pinpoint what needs to be done and how to do it, and we must develop a strategy of aid and development attractive to people everywhere and their governments, as well as the NGOs and private-sector funding sources that stand ready to assist in the achievement of this great goal. Right now it is the private sector working through the environmental nongovernmental organizations that forms the spearhead of the global conservation effort. The largest of these organizations working out of the United States (including Conservation International, the Nature Conservancy, and the World Wildlife Fund) have reached operating budgets at the $100 million level. They have enough influence now to form partnerships with the World Bank and the United Nations as well as work with the CEOs of larger corporations. They are backed by hundreds of smaller NGOs operating at levels from cities and countries to international venues. The NGOs are in general more entrepreneurial; they are more innovative and flexible than governments. But governments, at least those of industrialized countries, still do the heavy lifting, and will have to assume a larger role in the future. At the present time, about $6 billion a year is spent worldwide in conservation, proceeding from both private and governmental sources; most of this amount is ultimately from government sources.

Our recent estimates suggest that about $28 billion is needed to sustain much of the world's tropical ecosystems and a large part of the biodiversity within them.[10] We must keep in mind that this amount is only about one part in a thousand, or one-tenth of 1 percent, of the combined gross national products of the world. And we must also keep in mind that biodiversity represents a large part of our natural capital heritage—the Creation itself.

In this new century, as we attempt to find a solution to the problem of both raising standards of living in developing countries and saving the natural habitats in those same places, we should remember that the solution must flow from the recognition that each depends on the other. The poor, especially the nearly 1 billion people who are absolutely destitute, have little chance to improve their lives in a devastated environment. Conversely, the natural environments where most of biodiversity hangs on cannot survive the press of land-hungry people who have nowhere else to go.

This problem can be solved. We have the resources to accomplish it. And those who control those resources have many reasons to achieve that goal, not the least of which is their own security. At the end of the day, however, the direction we take will have to be an ethical decision. A civilization that can envision God and the afterlife and embark on the colonization of space will surely find the way to save the integrity of this magnificent planet and the life it harbors.

Notes

1. Sandra Postel, *Pillar of Sand: Can the Irrigation Miracle Last?* (New York: W.W. Norton, 1999).

2. Mathis Wackernagel, et al. *Living Planet Report 2000* (Gland, Switzerland: Worldwide Fund for Nature), pp. 10–12.

3. Fouad Ajami, *Foreign Policy* 119: 30–4 (Summer 2000).

4. In fact, one of the great frontiers of biology today is the exploration of microbial biodiversity and microbial ecology. Now, about 7,000 species of bacteria are formally recognized in the Bergey's manual, the official manual of species. But the earliest DNA diagnosis or sampling of bacterial species in soil indicates that nearly that number—4,000–5,000 species—will be found in one pinch of soil in a forest, or one pinch of marine sediment.

5. I believe that NASA has begun to study this species to help them consider what they might look for in terms of finding life on Mars.

6. There are various ingenious ways being developed to get to that canopy; rope-climbing is one popular way. Some French scientists have thought of another one: they lower a blimp, and then rappel down like a team of invading policemen and spread out over a cargo net suspended under the blimp. There is another method, developed in Panama by the Smithsonian Tropical Research Institute, which seems to be becoming the preferred method—*if* you can get the equipment. You bring in a building crane, hook up an investigator on the end of the crane, and lower him or her onto the canopy. You are probably thinking that we only make graduate students do this, but it's safer than it sounds; there is a gondola attached, complete with a screen that can be closed quickly to protect against the wasps and Africanized bees there.

7. Edward O. Wilson, *The Diversity of Life* (Cambridge, MA: Belknap Press of Harvard University Press, 1992).

8. William Newmark, *Conservation Biology* 9 (3): 512–26 (1995).

9. Edward O. Wilson, *The Future of Life* (New York: Knopf, 2001).

10. Ibid.

Part III

Racial Reconciliation:
Theory and Practice in America

United We Stand

Terrorism and National Identity

Angelika Bammer

The Blossoming of Flags

> *Flags are blossoming now where little else is blossoming and I am bent on fathoming what it means to love my country.*

—Adrienne Rich, "An Atlas of the Difficult World"

In the aftermath of what has come to be known in the United States as "9/11"—the terrorist attacks on the World Trade Center, the Pentagon, and the foiled attack on a third target, perhaps the White House, that took place in the morning hours of September 11, 2001—flags, American flags, were everywhere. People wore them, attached them to their mailboxes, houses, and cars, and decorated yards and windows, grocery and laundry bags with them. They even showed up on baby pacifiers. And this display of flags has remained ever-present ever since as part of our everyday landscape. What are these flags about? Whom are they speaking to and for? And how are we to read their mute, insistent repetition?

As Sigmund Freud observes in *Beyond the Pleasure Principle*, the experience of repetition—the re-experiencing of something identical—is often a source of pleasure, providing the reassurance of the familiar, the aesthetic satisfaction of discovering patterns. But it can also be the opposite, a source of *un*pleasure, imparting the feeling of being stuck, of repetition without progress, of not being able to move on. Our memories of the past are both pleasurable and painful in just these ways: memories we call up can recollect happy times—times of confidence, optimism, or joy—just as memories that come up, unsummoned, can pull us back to psychic spaces we would just as soon forget or leave behind. These latter, Freud notes, are memories of the unresolved past that linger in our psyche like unbid guests who will not leave. Ghostly presences that shadow our unconscious everyday, offering neither resolution nor solace, they are inaccessible to our conscious grasp. And so we keep going back to them in our minds, as unable to get rid of them as we are to fully claim them. As Freud put it, such pleasureless and unproductive returns are compulsive, not willed. And this compulsion to repeat, he explained, is frequently a manifestation of trauma.

In this essay I draw on Freud's opposition between productive remembering and unproductive repetition to attempt a reading of the proliferation of American flags in the post-9/11 cultural landscape. I propose that these flags signify both positive (in Freud's sense of pleasureful, i.e., confident, assertive, proud) and negative (in Freud's sense of *un*pleasureful, i.e., fearful, angry, confused) responses to the terrorist attacks, and that the doubledness of this response reveals a profound ambivalence at the heart of contemporary Americans' sense of nation. In particular, I will suggest that in their astonishing abundance, these flags might be read as a sign of deep uncertainty about the meaning and condition of the very national unity that they, in their manifest symbolism, are supposed to affirm.

On the most explicit and immediately recognizable level, of course, the flags were a show of pride and strength, a strength deployed as much by the routine business conducted in and around the very area where the now destroyed World Trade Center towers had stood, as by the Air Force jets that were soon to roar over Afghanistan, dropping bombs. As quintessential symbols of national identity and reminders of American power, the flags were an assertive response to an outside threat, a forceful expression of national resolve. And this resolve, the flags in their ubiquity and sameness seemed to suggest, was unified. It spoke with a single voice.

This unity, and the strength derived from it, was directly related to the trauma that the nation as a whole had just experienced. For, as the French historian Ernest Renan had posited in his landmark essay, "What Is a Nation?," the very ability of people to speak, and to experience themselves, as a people, grows out of their shared memory not of glory, but of pain. Writing in 1882, barely a decade after the brutal end of the Franco-Prussian War, which left a vanquished and humiliated French nation to sign off on its own defeat in the royal palace of Versailles, the people in its capital starving, Renan declared that what binds a people together as a nation is not who they are in some originary sense (a common race, people joined by bloodlines or by the same native language), but what they have become in the course of the memories they share of experiences undergone and activities undertaken together. Obviously, this includes the "great deeds" they as a people have performed together, as well as the "wish to perform still more" (Renan 1990/1882, 19). But, Renan continues, even more than these, even more than the "glorious heritage" of a "heroic past, great men, [and] glory," and, "in the future, [a shared] programme to put into effect," it is "the sacrifices to which one has consented . . . the ills that one has suffered"—in short, as he puts it, the "regrets"—that, in the end, forge a nation. "[S]uffering in common," he declares, "unifies more than joy does." Therefore, Renan concludes, "[w]here national memories are concerned, griefs are of more value than triumphs."

Griefs are of more value than triumphs, to repeat Renan, for eminently practical reasons: "they impose duties and require a common effort" (Renan 1990/1882, 19). In the American aftermath of September 11, 2001, the shared grief and the common effort that devolved from it were unmistakable. To ask what suffering we had in common as a people at that time would, to most, have seemed ludicrous. The injury was clear. We had all experienced it in some way. Seared into our mind's eyes were images of airplanes full of passengers exploding into skyscrapers over one hundred stories high, bodies falling from the sky like birds on fire, giant buildings collapsing in clouds of ash. And, when the dust had settled and the flames subsided, we lived with the memory of close to three thousand people dead, their bodies forever lost under over a million tons of rubble rising up to fifty feet high in the heart of New York City. The flags were an immediate and spontaneous response to the shock of this devastation, an assertion that, even in the face of such violation and numbing loss, we held strong and "stood united." In this regard, as an expression of unity and resolve, the display of flags that was repeated over and over again, on all sides, was a deliberate act of collective will.

But if we read the repetition of post-9/11 flags less as a willed *response* to collective trauma than as a much less conscious *manifestation* of a traumatic experience, then their meaning is less self-evident. Clearly, they signify something about nation, for "nation" is what flags officially represent. However, instead of seeing the ubiquitous American flags as expressions of American-ness, as if the meaning of "America" were clear, we could also see them as an attempt to interrogate what "America" meant to Americans as a people at this time. As Susan Willis points out in her reflections on the flag in a collection of post-9/11 essays, the very dissemenation of the American flag in the aftermath of the terrorist attacks resulted in a corresponding proliferation of meanings. The flag, in other words, came to mean many different things, depending on the context. It could "generate certain specific meanings in its New York incarnation," Willis notes, "and very different ones over Kandahar," or, we might add, Atlanta or Detroit (Willis 2002, 377). Paradoxically, Willis continues, it was this very signifying emptiness that charged the flag with supersymbolic power, compounding, as it circulated, a volatile brew of everyday patriotism, nationalist militarism, capitalist consumerism, and politicized evangelicism. Politically speaking, I quite agree. However, what Willis's political analysis leaves out is the fact that the very instability and emptiness of this supercharged flag symbol enabled it to signify both positive and negative at once: *both* an assertive belief in American might and right *and* anxiety about their loss or diminution. Indeed, psychoanalytically speaking, from the perspective of compulsive repetition as a sign of trauma, one could see the ubiquitous flags less as an expression of Americans' confidence and strength than as a manifestation of their heightened state of uncertainty and fear. If this is so, then fear of what?

Answers to this question were quick and ready at hand, seemingly as obvious as the nature of the trauma from which it stemmed. We were afraid, we were told, of those who had harmed us and would again, who had attacked and continued to threaten us. We rehearsed fear of those named as our enemies in this respect: people from foreign countries with foreign values and foreign names: Osama bin Laden, al-Qaeda, "Arabs," "the Muslim world," "them." And, in response to this identification of what we were told that we feared, the military was mobilized to seal our borders, patrol our skies, and watch over us. To protect "us," we had to keep "them" out.

However, the problem with this solution, conceptually and practically, was right away obvious: "they" were not just outside, foreign enemies "over there." They were here. In fact, "they" were inseparable from "us": neighbors, colleagues, friends of our children, members of our families. What is more, "they" frequently, literally, *were* us in our various states of hybrid identities, multiple affiliations, and divided loyalties. The truth was that, in the confusing maelstrom of the 9/11 crisis, while we indeed often found ourselves afraid or suspicious of those defined as "them," we also, as a people, found ourselves confronting the even more disturbing fact that, perhaps even more than "them," what we really feared was ourselves.

A clue to this fact lay in another set of ritualized gestures that often accompanied the flags: the repeated proclamations on decals, bumper stickers, yard signs, and, in the immediate aftermath of the attacks, even television ticker tape scrolls, that declared "we stand united." The claim itself, in its familiarity, was relatively unremarkable, but the degree of its repetition was not. This repetition, similarly compulsive in its rote application as the accompanying display of flags, suggests that perhaps another trauma had come into play that was not defined by—or as—foreign terrorism. Perhaps the continual affirmation that we stood united was, in fact, a clue to a fear that we could not yet even consciously admit, a fear about the state of our very unitedness itself. This fear was not of others and the harm they might do to us, but of ourselves and the consequences of the harm we routinely inflict on one another, particularly on those of us marked as different in some way. For, despite the assurance repeated endlessly in those tense weeks and months after September 11 that our diversity was our strength, our history reminded us that this assurance was a very fragile bridge over chasms of pain and rage-filled differences. And we knew, from our history and the reminder we had just received, that under pressure those differences could explode as suddenly and unexpectedly as an act of terror on a sunny, blue-sky day.

Perhaps this, then, is another way to understand the ubiquitous flags: as an expression of fear that we, as a people, might not be up to the challenge of the very unity we so proudly and loudly proclaimed. Could a people as deeply divided as we were—in our cultural roots, our material realities, our spiritual strivings, and our political goals—join together to form a national community that would hold? Perhaps the insistence that "we stand united" revealed a deeper fear that the flags, in their patriotic symbolism, masked, namely the fear that, under pressure, we might just fracture along the fault lines of our differences, not standing united, but facing off.

The tremors along these fault lines reverberate across the arenas of national and international politics, particularly in times of stress. But they also reverberate in the most quotidian and mundane interactions within local communities and personal relationships. This was brought home to me around the time of the first 9/11 anniversary, when I went to find our winter coats. They were in the back closet, where we had hung them in the spring, still wrapped in the plastic bags from the dry cleaner's. What startled me, perhaps because I had not noticed it at the time, perhaps because in our household national symbols show up rather rarely, was the design on the plastic bags: a large red, white, and blue American flag and, beneath it, the caption "America United." The next time I went to our local dry cleaners, I asked them about these bags. They knew them well, although now, a good year later, they were not using them anymore. "After 9/11," said the young Pakistani woman who co-owns the business with her brother, "the supplier added them to the order forms. And we ordered them: laundry bags, hangers, business cards . . . "All with flags?" I asked. "All with flags." "We love America," her brother, who had been listening in on our conversation, burst in. "We love America."

What, I wondered, did this declaration mean? Obviously, it could be taken, simply and directly, at face value, a declaration of allegiance to this country in which we—they and I and some of our family—lived. Yet, perhaps in part because I myself am foreign-born, I could not help but think that the emphatic nature of the declaration might also have something to do with the fact that most of the dry cleaning franchises in our community are owned by Indians or Pakistanis, people who, because of their dark skin and "foreign" accents, have often, particularly after 9/11, been taken for foreigners from "over there," their actual citizenship notwithstanding. From this perspective, the dry cleaners' declaration of allegiance to America and their very visible display of American flags could be as much a sign of patriotism as of a perceived outsider's feelings of vulnerability.

Who, "We"?

Some years ago, a joke circulated in progressive circles that was designed to remind us of the unstable, situationally shifting, nature of "us" and "them" identifications. The joke came in different versions; I heard it as the one about the Lone Ranger and his trusty sidekick, Tonto. As usual, they are out riding together, the white man leading and the Indian at his side. Tonto, trained in scouting, sees a party of Indians coming at them in full war gear. He signals their approach to the Lone Ranger. "Indians! Tonto, we're in trouble!" the Lone Ranger cries. Tonto shrugs and looks at the Lone Ranger and back at the Indians and smiles, "What do you mean, we, white man?"

The truth is, we are never a unitary and hardly ever a stable "we." We are divided within and among ourselves. In times of stress the divisions simply become more palpable. These truths apply to nations also. As the political historian Benedict Anderson has argued in his landmark study of how people come to think of themselves as a nation—how people become *a people*—there is nothing natural or given about such entities. A people are a nation because, as Anderson famously put it, they *imagine* themselves to be. As they do things that enact and ritually symbolize this "imagined community," like consume the same news, grieve the same losses, or fly the same flag, a nation in the form of this imagined community takes hold. However, in a sense, it never really, materially, exists: it remains a postulate, a wager, a promise, an act of faith. We re-create it every day. And in so doing we realize how tenuous and fragile it actually is, particularly in times of danger.

Those perceived as "Other"—as the "them" to our "us"—are seen as threats to this sense of community. "We," by definition, are the ones who belong; "they" don't, by the same definition.

Therefore, as the sociologist Zygmunt Baumann explains, the relationship between "us" and "them" is structured as opposition: the one is "the group to which I belong" and the other the "group to which I either cannot or do not wish to belong" (Baumann 1990, 40). Within my group, I thus feel "secure and at home," while "they" appear hostile and frightening. As Baumann puts it, "I expect them . . . to act against my interests, to seek to do me harm and bring me misfortune" and, when they have done so, "to rejoice in my misery" (40–41).

The structural paradox, however, is that, even as we oppose each other, we need each other in equal measure. The very solidarity, mutual trust, and loyalty by which we believe in and know ourselves as "us," are based on our ability to know, with equal certainty, that we are definitely not "them." In fact, we are "us" precisely because we are not "them." Our mutual otherness is the guarantor of our respective group identities. As Baumann explains it, using the sociological categories of in-group versus out-group, "an out-group is precisely that imaginary opposition to itself which the in-group needs for its self-identity, for its cohesiveness, for its inner solidarity and emotional security" (41–42). "[W]ere there no such group," he concludes, "it would have to be invented." For, structurally speaking, "they" do not threaten "us," but rather are constitutive of our us-ness.

There are, however, others who *do* threaten us in our secure and bounded feeling of us-ness, and they do so precisely because they cannot be contained in either an in-group or out-group structure. These are the people whom Baumann describes as "strangers": "neither close nor distant. Neither a part of 'us' nor a part of 'them.' Neither friends nor foes" (1990, 55). They do not hold to the established boundaries. And so, they confuse us and cause anxiety, as we "do not know exactly what . . . to make of them, what to expect, how to behave" (55). For their status is unclear: they are ambiguous. And thus Baumann explains in structural terms what we know experientially, namely that, often more than outright antagonism, which can reassure us with its positional clarity, it is ambiguity that we find threatening. Susan Willis, in her analysis of the politics of American patriotism, concurs, citing Americans' "deep cultural antipathy for ambiguity" as the foundation of their cultural ethos that every problem can be fixed and that it is they who must do the fixing. The insistence that all the bodies of all of those who have disappeared or been destroyed in disasters such as the 9/11 attacks must be recovered and positively identified is but one example, she notes, of this peculiarly American insistence on and "desperate desire" for closure (Willis 2002, 381).What Willis sees critically, as a national form of social pathology, Baumann sees structurally, as an expression of people's need to constitute binding communities. Ambiguity, he reasons, is threatening because it leaves the boundaries between "us" and "them" open and undefined and thus, in the end, indefensible.

What is more, Baumann points out, in light of this ambiguity, we begin to doubt ourselves. For, rather than fortify our sense of who we are in the act of defending ourselves against an enemy, those who are both "us" and "not us"—dissidents, heretics, traitors, deserters, renegades, newcomers, immigrants, refugees, interlopers—undermine our very ability to assert or affirm ourselves (Baumann 1990, 58). For what we take as given is not self-evident to them, and to them, many of our most hallowed certainties can seem strange. As a result, in our encounters with them, we often find ourselves forced to question ourselves in ways that threaten both our sense of security and our sense of confidence. They make us uncomfortable. And that scares us. And being scared makes us angry.

The eighteenth-century moral philosopher and social theorist Adam Smith explains the discomfort caused by those whom Baumann has termed "strangers" as a lack of what he calls "fellow-feeling." Fellow-feeling, as Smith sees it, is generated by the sympathy we feel for another whom we experience, or imagine, to be like us. It occurs spontaneously and, as Smith puts it, "naturally" (Smith 1976/1795, 10). And yet this natural impulse has a critical social function. For it is the emotional glue that holds a social body together, "the active binding agency of collective life" (Herbert 1991, 83). Moreover, Smith argues, this fellow-feeling is not only psychological, it is also ethical. For it both determines how a person *feels* about another and frames the way we see, understand, and judge of one another: "Every faculty in one man is the measure by which he judges of the like faculty in another. I judge of your sight by my sight, of your ear by my ear, of your reason by my reason, of your resentment by my resentment, of your love by my love. I neither have, nor can have, any other way of judging about them" (Smith, 19).

In his model of social memory, the British social scientist Paul Connerton offers an explanation for the apparent naturalness of Smith's notion of fellow-feeling. A society constitutes itself, he proposes, by continuing to re-enact its own remembrance of itself, and this re-enactment of social memory is not only organized in the form of public commemorative ceremonies, it is also incorporated into the most unconscious, and thus seemingly natural, details of bodily practices: how and when we sit, stand, rise, bow our heads, avert our eyes, cry, blush, or smile. These mnemonics of the body, to put it in Connerton's terms, embed social memory deeply into an infinite number of privately enacted, but collectively recognized and ritually repeated, daily events. As such, this bodily "habit-memory" powerfully undergirds the cohesion and stability of our social structures. We recognize who "we" are by doing basic things the way "we" do them. And, in the continual process of such recognitions and repetitions, we reconstitute ourselves communally in our own likeness, generating and spreading vital fellow-feeling among ourselves. Therefore, Connerton concludes, a social pluralism model based on diversity poses much greater challenges to social stability than an assimilation model based on sameness, as the admission of difference undermines the notion that the habit-memory we have incorporated is natural, rather than learned. Those whose bodily practices exhibit a different social memory from ours thus make us uncomfortable in ways that we feel personally, but understand socially. In their presence, we do not feel as fully, i.e., un-self-consciously, at home anymore.

Not *feeling* at home, even though we *are* at home, is an experience that psychoanalysis has described as "uncanny." *Unheimlich*—the German term rendered in English as "uncanny"—means, literally, "unhomely." Over a decade before Freud's famous exploration of this phenomenon in his essay "The Uncanny," a colleague of his, the pathologist and psychologist Ernst Jentsch, had already described the uncanny as the experience of not feeling quite "'at home' or 'at ease'" (Jentsch 1995/1906, 8). He describes it as a state of "psychical uncertainty" and observes that it is often related to the presence of those whom Baumann would call "strangers." For, as Jentsch notes, a typical instance of such a state, commonly observed among "primitive" peoples, is a "wariness in relation to unusual people, who think otherwise, feel differently, and act otherwise than the majority" (10). Put another way, we are more likely to feel psychologically "not at home" in the presence of those with whom we don't share fellow-feeling. And, as Adam Smith points out in his discussion of fellow-feeling, its absence can make a relationship impossible or intolerable: "if you have either no fellow-feeling for the misfortunes I have met with, or none that bears any proportion to the grief which distracts me; or if you have either no indignation at the injuries I have suffered, or none that bears any proportion to the resentment which transports me, we can no longer converse upon these subjects. We become intolerable to one another" (Smith 1976/1795, 21).

If "we can no longer converse" or have "become intolerable to one another," what do we do? We blame it on the others, observes Jentsch, and we produce an explanation that enables us to restore the feeling of comfort we think they took from us. This explanation, notes Jentsch, need not be true in the sense of "based on fact." What matters, rather, is that it enable us to dispel the "awkward affect"—the feeling ill at ease—by attributing it to others. Such a repositioning of the source of the problem provides the "psychical shelter" we need (Jentsch 1995/1906, 15). Paul Connerton corroborates as a social scientist what Jentsch observes as a psychologist. Connerton, too, notes that our typical response to the discomfort we experience in the presence of others who are different from ourselves is to conclude that they have done something wrong or are in the wrong place. If we are ill at ease, it must be they who caused it.

But, as the Lacanian-trained social theorist and post-Marxian philosopher Slavoj Zizek points out, in blaming our discomfort on the others, we have it exactly wrong: the problem with the others is not the others, but ourselves. For while we say that we do not want to deal with "them" anymore, we actually are quite obsessed with them. They are, as one might put it in Lacanian psychoanalytic terms, the objects of our desire. We are fascinated by their very otherness because it represents precisely what we do not—and cannot logically ever—have: the experience of being not-us. Given this impossibility, we fantasize that "they" have the very qualities we lack—greater power, less pain, and, above all, more pleasure—and we cannot stop wanting whatever we think it is they have. In this sense, Zizek points out, the Other is not real, an actual other person, but the fantasized representation of an imagined lack within ourselves, a fear of something missing, incomplete. And for that reason we want to hurt them: not because they have actually done something to us or taken something away, but because their sheer presence—the mere fact of their being Other—takes away from us the perhaps most precious thing of all: the illusion that we are complete within ourselves.

One response to this problem is to make these Others disappear by ignoring them, segregating them, evicting them, or, finally, killing them, even if we, in our obsessive fascination with them, end up destroying ourselves in the process. This is the horror of the very logic that Jean Baudrillard unfolds in his post-9/11 reflections on "the spirit of terrorism." Reflecting on terrorism and the relationship between "us" and "them" in the context of American global hegemony, Baudrillard takes Zizek's notion of the Other as the fantasized object of our desire and turns it on its head: *we*, he proposes, are the object of the *others'* envious desire. But then, he points out, since "we," as a global hegemon, have virtually incorporated all the others within our imperial reach, we end up *becoming* them in our own fantasy of ourselves, as we think that they must see us. In this sense, as he puts it, power, dispersed globally and exercised hegemonically, becomes "complicitous in its own destruction" (Baudrillard 2002, 13; my translation).[1] And so, Baudrillard reaches the chilling conclusion that "they" only did what "we" actually wanted to do ourselves, namely destroy ourselves in a frenzy of annihilationist envy. "Put in the most extreme way," he concludes, "it is they who did it, but we who wanted it done" (11; my translation).[2]

Force and Its Alternatives

Baudrillard's argument notwithstanding, violence—getting rid of those we perceive as Other—does not relieve us of discomfort. For, as Zizek proposes, these very Others, in their constitutive otherness, are the prod-

ucts of our fantasies, projections of our own desires that have gone un-
satisfied. They are, in that sense, ourselves. Yard signs that have been
sprouting up across American neighborhoods of late translate this psychological recognition into political terms to conclude that "War Is Not
the Answer."

It is a year and a winter after the events of 9/11 and we are gearing up
for war. Flags are still up, although they are fading now, not new. The
yard signs against war are more recent. Taken together, the convergence
of flags and signs marks a significant change in our political landscape.
For in the mute dialogue between the red, white, and blue flags and the
blue, dove-emblemed signs, any sense of a unified, national voice has
disappeared. The very things that, in the immediate aftermath of 9/11,
had seemed clear enough to all are now manifestly in question: what we
stand for or oppose, what makes us feel threatened or secure, and whether,
in the face of a potential war, we can—and want to—stand united.

These are the very kind of questions asked in a famous exchange of
public letters between Albert Einstein and Sigmund Freud in the early
1930s, at a time when the specter of war that had shadowed Europe
since the uneasy resolution of World War I was looming larger and drawing closer. In response to this growing sense of impending threat, the
League of Nations, through the International Institute of Intellectual
Cooperation, organized an international series of open letters between
public intellectuals who supported its general goals. Einstein was one of
the first to be approached; he agreed to participate and suggested Freud
as his interlocutor. Freud agreed. Their letters were written in 1932:
Einstein wrote Freud from Potsdam in July; Freud responded from Vienna
in September. The letters were published in Paris in 1933—the year that
Hitler came to power as the elected leader of the German government—
as volume two of the International Institute's open letter series. The title
was, *Warum Krieg? Pourquoi la guerre? Why War?*[3]

Einstein poses the initial question: Is there a way to prevent war?[4]
His conclusion is pessimistic, as he enumerates the obstacles: nation-
states are reluctant to empower a supranational body with the authority
to prevent them from pursuing their own interests, including the right to
wage war; unscrupulous groups are always eager and ready to profit
from the commerce of war; and people in general seem driven by "a
need to hate and destroy" (Einstein and Freud 1964/1933, 19; my translation).[5] The problem, in short, is that "right and might are inseparable,"
as Einstein notes, and that those with the power to determine right are

usually those with the most unchecked hold on might (15; my translation).[6] Freud's response takes up from there. Noting the slippery and ambiguous meaning of the term *power* (*Macht*), his first move is an attempt at clarification. "May I replace the word 'power' with the harsher, harder word 'violence'?" he thus begins (27; my translation).[7] And with this simple lexical switch, he exposes the dimension of force obscured by power's semantic ambiguity. Power, notes Freud, *is*, in essence, force that, if resisted, will turn to violence.[8] It can only lose this dimension of force if it moves from the exclusivity of individual control to be shared among people communally. For, as he explains, this is the shift that enables power (*Macht*) to become law (*Recht*). However, he goes on, even shared power enacted as law is based on force and the threat of violence, as long as the community in question feels threatened in any way, either internally or from the outside. Thus, force—relentlessly and, if need be, violently imposed—is what ensures that the community will hold together.

There is, grants Freud, another option in place of force to secure the bonds that form community: the development of "affective ties . . . between its members" (Einstein and Freud, 1964/1933, 41; my translation).[9] For that reason, he concludes, in the end, the only way to prevent war (or, one might add, internal violence) is to develop and nurture such affective ties within and among communities. As he puts it, "[a]nything that produces affective ties between people necessarily works to counter war" (53; my translation).[10] The problem is that these affective ties are not necessarily affectionate. "Love thy neighbor as thyself" is, Freud acknowledges, easier said than done. A more achievable goal is the kind of connection that results from people recognizing and acknowledging interests they share through a process of identification as an interest group (*Interessengemeinschaft*). For, Freud posits, the process of acknowledging shared interests and identifying in this way invariably results in the development of affective ties and what Adam Smith called "fellow-feeling."[11] In other words, shared interests and the readiness for joint action need not *originate in* fellow-feeling, as if commonalty simply followed from who we are. The reverse is just as likely, perhaps more. A recognition of shared interests and the resulting readiness for joint action also *leads to* a feeling of connectedness among those whom a sense of shared purpose has brought together. For, Freud explains, the affective ties on which social community is based are seldom, if ever, natural. They are rather, in the manner of the kind of community they produce, themselves social: shaped by a sense of common cause. Indeed, he concludes, it is not *natural feelings of liking*, but rather *deliberate and pragmatic identifications of common interests* that structurally undergird human society and enable it to function.

With this conclusion, Freud returns to an earlier point in his thoughts on the question of war and human society that Einstein's letter of July 1932 had raised, namely an essay that he had written in the spring of 1915, several months after the outbreak of World War I.[12] It was published that same year, in conjunction with a reflection on human attitudes toward death, as Reflections on War and Death ("Zeitgemasses uber Krieg und Tod").[13] In this essay, Freud does not begin with moral censure on the order of "war is wrong," but rather with the psychological observation that "war is disappointing." Why is war, as he puts it, "disappointing"? Because, he explains, "we"—we, who had thought of ourselves as "the great ruling nations of the white race, the leaders of mankind, who had cultivated world wide interests, and to whom we owe the technical progress in the control of nature as well as the creation of artistic and scientific cultural standards," we, who as heirs of the Enlightenment had "acquired sufficient understanding for the qualities . . . [people] had in common and enough tolerance for their differences so that . . . the words 'foreign' and 'hostile' should no longer be synonymous"—we had revealed ourselves, to ourselves and to the entire world, to be barbarous, crude, "uncivilized" (Freud 1918, 4 and 6). Instead of finding "some other way of settling . . . differences and conflicting interests," we had reverted to violence and gone to war against those we had branded as "foreign" and, therefore, "hostile." The disappointment of war, he thus concludes, "consists in the destruction of an illusion": the illusion that we were somehow better than we actually were (6).

But "better" and "worse" are moral categories that do not take into account either psychological or social factors. Psychologically speaking, we are driven by impulses that are "in themselves neither good nor evil," Freud points out, and, socially speaking, we are compelled, not by conscience, but by "social fear" (Freud 1918, 15).[14] And civilization— the ability to behave better than we actually feel on the level of our primal impulses—rests on our willingness to temper the solipsism of selfish want with the restraint of social fear. It rests, as Freud puts it, on our ability to transform "selfish impulses into social impulses" (21).[15] In other words, in the balance between "living according to the psychological truth" and a "civilized hypocrisy" that bends our selfish impulses to accommodate social needs, it is the latter, in the end, that is preferable. Indeed, Freud concludes, probably "a certain amount of civilized hyprocrisy [*Kulturheuchelei*] is . . . indispensable to maintain civilization" (1918, 28–29). "Civilized hypocrisy," then, rather than "living according to the truth," provides the basis for the creation of the kind of affective ties that can hold a community together without the use or threat of force.

"Civilized hypocrisy" means accepting an inherently compromised state on the grounds that such compromise makes it possible to tolerate differences that may, on an impulse level, seem intolerable. In short, tolerance—the very foundation of civilization, as Freud notes—is invariably bought at a psychological cost. Ernst Jentsch, a decade earlier, had reached a similar conclusion, noting that if we want to accommodate the presence of people "who think otherwise, feel differently, and act otherwise" than ourselves, we must accept the fact that "we" live in a social space that is not ours alone, but shared with others. This is not easy: it requires the willingness to make sacrifices and endure discomfort. Above all, it takes work. For, as Adam Smith points out in the chapter on "sympathy" with which *The Theory of Moral Sentiments* begins, if "fellow-feeling" does not come naturally, out of sympathy between you and me—if there is, in short, a "want of feeling"—we must *work* ("endeavor . . . and strive," in Smith's words) to imagine a shared state upon which sympathy could be fashioned (Smith 1976/1795, 21).

Paradoxically, the hardest work of all might even be to not do anything: to *not* act, rather than rush impulsively toward given ends; to undo assumptions or fixed notions in order to allow space and time in which to consider—and reconsider—a given situation and our response. Such work—the work of waiting, of taking care and pulling back—is, as the poet Ingeborg Bachman points out, hard for many reasons: it goes unnoticed and unrewarded, and it is unending: "every day."[16] If there is any reward for such work, she suggests, it is, at best, "the modest star of hope" that we can pin on "[t]he uniform of the day . . . patience" (Bachmann 1986/1978, 103). Thus prepared, dressed in patience and with "hope upon the heart," we might perhaps be able to begin imagining the kind of people and communities we could be if we were willing to replace the power of force with the power of affective ties, ties grounded in the simple and awesome willingness to live as human beings together.

Notes

1. "Elle [la puissance] est complice de sa propre destruction." I am quoting from the French original of Baudrillard's essay, *L'esprit du terrorisme*, which first appeared in the French newspaper *Le monde* in November 2001 and was published by Galilee as a separate volume in 2002. The English translation has added a second essay, "Requiem for the Twin Towers," which Baudrillard first presented in a debate on the events of September 11, 2001, and their effects held in New York City in February 2002.

2. " . . . c'est eux qui l'ont fait, mais c'est nous qui l'avons voulu."

3. Subsequent references are to this original publication; where noted, I have given my own translation of the German original. The original 1933 version of this correspondence in English was translated by Stuart Gilbert. In *The Standard Edition of the Complete Psychological Works of Sigmund Freud*, the Gilbert translation of Einstein's letter is unchanged, while Freud's letter has been re-translated by James Strachey.

4. In his formulation: "Gibt es einen Weg, die Menschen von dem Verhangnis des Krieges zu befreien?" (Einstein and Freud 1933, 12). The Gilbert translation puts this as, "Is there any way of delivering mankind from the menace of war?" (Einstein and Freud 1964/1933, 199).

5. "Im Menschen lebt ein Bedürfnis zu hassen und zu vernichten." The Gilbert translation puts this as, "man has within him a lust for hatred and destruction" (Einstein and Freud 1964/1933, 201).

6. "Recht und Macht sind unzertrennlich verbunden." The German *Macht* could also be translated as "power," in this case. Indeed, the discussion between Einstein and Freud deliberately works with the semantic ambiguity of the German terms *Recht* (which means both "law" and "right") and *Macht* (which means both "power" and "might") to stage the slippage between public and personal forms of right, psychological and social forms of power. This ambiguity and slippage gets lost in the need to choose between discrete lexical terms in English.

7. "Darf ich das Wort 'Macht' durch das grellere, härtere Wort 'Gewalt' ersetzen?"

8. The German word *Gewalt* connotes both "force" and "violence."

9. "Die Gefühlsbindungen der Mitglieder."

10. "Alles, was Gefuhlsbindungen unter den Menschen herstellt, muss dem Krieg entgegenwirken."

11. Freud's term for affective ties of this kind is "feelings of community" (*Gemeinschaftsgefuhle*) (Einstein and Freud 1964/1933, 33). The Strachey translation renders this as "communal feelings."

12. The German title of this essay is "Die Enttauschung des Krieges." In the *Standard Edition* of Freud's works, edited by James Strachey, it is translated as "The Disillusionment of the War." In the initial (1918) English translation by Alfred Brill and Alfred Kuttner, it was rendered as "The Disappointments of War." I prefer the latter's lexical choice for its emphasis on the emotional ("disappointment")—as compared to the intellectual ("disillusionment")—impact of the war that Freud reflects on in this essay. Thus, my references are to the earlier edition.

13. The initial Brill and Kuttner translation, *Reflections on War and Death*, of 1918 was subsequently replaced by a new translation, "Thoughts for the Times on War and Death," by E. C. Mayne; this latter has become the standard English rendering of Freud's text.

14. "Social fear" (*soziale Angst*) is both italicized and in quotation marks in the German original.

15. At the same time, Freud reminds us that we necessarily *begin* with primal selfishness. Indeed, as he notes, "[t]he most pronounced childish egotists may become the most helpful and self-sacrificing citizens; the majority of idealists, humanitarians, and protectors of animals have developed from little sadists and animal tormentors" (Freud 1918, 21).

16. "Every day" ("*Alle Tage*") is the central poem in Bachmann's 1953 poetry collection, *Die gestundete Zeit* (Deferred Time); it was first presented in a radio broadcast in November 1952.

Bibliography

Anderson, Benedict. 1991. *Imagined Communities: Reflections on the Origin and Spread of Nationalism*. Rev. ed. London and New York: Verso.

Bachmann, Ingeborg. 1986/1978. "Every Day" [Alle Tage]. Translated by Kate Flores. In *The Defiant Muse: German Feminist Poems from the Middle Ages to the Present. A Bilingual Anthology*, 102–105, ed. Susan L. Cocalis. New York: The Feminist Press.

Baudrillard, Jean. 2002. *L'esprit du terrorisme*. Paris: Galilée. [English translation by Chris Turner. *The Spirit of Terrorism, and Requiem for the Twin Towers*. London and New York: Verso, 2002.

Baumann, Zygmunt. 1990. *Thinking Sociologically*. Oxford, UK, and Cambridge, MA: Blackwell.

Einstein, Albert, and Sigmund Freud. 1964/1933. *Warum Krieg?* [English translation by Stuart Gilbert (Einstein letter) and James Strachey (Freud letter)."Why War?" In *The Standard Edition of the Complete Psychological Works of Sigmund Freud*. Vol. 22, 197–215. London: The Hogarth Press and the Institute of Psycho-Analysis, 1964.]

Freud, Sigmund. 1955/1920. *Beyond the Pleasure Principle*. Translated by James Strachey in collaboration with Anna Freud. *The Standard Edition of the Complete Psychological Works of Sigmund Freud*. Vol. 18. London: The Hogarth Press and the Institute of Psycho-Analysis. [Originally published as *Jenseits des Lustprinzips*. Leipzig, Vienna, and Zurich: Internationaler Psychoanalytischer Verlag, 1920.]

———. 1918. *Reflections on War and Death*. Translated by A.A. Brill and Alfred B. Kuttner. New York: Moffat, Yard and Company. [The more commonly referenced edition of this essay is "Thoughts for the Times on War and Death." Translated by James Strachey. In *The Standard Edition of the Complete Psychological Works of Sigmund Freud*. Vol. 14, 274–300. London: The Hogarth Press and the Institute of Psycho-Analysis. [The German original was published as "Zeitgemässes über Krieg und Tod." *Imago*, vol. 4, no. 1 (1915): 1–21.]

Herbert, Christopher. 1991. *Culture and Anomie: Ethnographic Imagination in the Nineteenth Century*. Chicago: University of Chicago Press.

Jentsch, Ernst. 1995/1906. "On the Psychology of the Uncanny." *Angelaki* 2.1: 7–16.

Renan, Ernest. 1990/1882. "What Is a Nation?" Translated by Martin Thom. In *Nation and Narration*, 8–22, ed. by Homi Bhabha. London and New York: Routledge.

Rich, Adrienne. 1991. "An Atlas of the Difficult World." In *An Atlas of the Difficult World: Poems 1998–1991*, 1–26. New York and London: W.W. Norton.

Smith, Adam. 1976/1795. *Theory of Moral Sentiments*. Oxford, England: Clarendon Press.

Strachey, James. 1964. "Editor's Note. *Warum Krieg?*" In *The Standard Edition of the Complete Psychological Works of Sigmund Freud*. Vol. 22. London: The Hogarth Press and the Institute of Psycho-Analysis.

Willis, Susan. 2002. "Old Glory." *South Atlantic Quarterly* 101:2 (Spring). Special edition, *Dissent from the Homeland: Essays After September 11*, edited by Stanley Hauerwar and Frank Lentricchia: 375–83.

Zizek, Slavoj. 1993. "Enjoy Your Nation as Yourself!" In *Tarrying with the Negative: Kant, Hegel, and the Critique of Ideology*, 200–85. Durham: Duke University Press.

Reconciliation and the Beloved Community

John Lewis

When I speak of reconciliation, I mean the ancient cry for peace and understanding. It is a cry as old as the dawn of civilization and as fresh as the rise of the sun. I can think of no better topic to address at this time in our history. Over the past few years, we have witnessed dramatic events in our nation and around the world: hunger, disease, revolution, and strife between people over religious beliefs and political doctrines. There is no better time than the present to talk about reconciliation and no better place to begin than with the vision of the beloved community.

In the beloved community we find compassion for others and justice for all. In the beloved community, we find a community at peace with itself, a community that must come together for the common good. In my vision of the beloved community, we are reconciled. We are brought together under one house—the American house, the American family. And even beyond the shores of our great country there is a world community sorely in need of unity and freedom from struggle. Without reconciliation, there can be no unity, there can be no beloved community. Some might say that this is an impossible dream held by a few aging hippies, peaceniks, and old, tired civil rights workers like myself. But there is no doubting that the America we see today is dramatically different from the America of my youth.

As a child of the South, my early years were spent in rural Alabama—then a setting of social, economic, and political servitude akin to slavery. My parents were enslaved by a system of tenant farming called sharecropping. They sweated over the land from sunup to sundown, and received very little for their labor. The world I knew as a child was divided in two—one black and the other white. In the 1940s and 1950s, I tasted the bitter fruits of segregation, racial discrimination, and prejudice. I saw those signs that separated people based on the color of their skin—white men, colored men, white women, colored women, white waiting, and colored waiting. I was bused to school long distances on unpaved roads that were dusty in the summer and muddy in the winter. The school I attended was poorly staffed, underheated, and segregated. We read from tattered books that were worn out because they had been used by students at the all-white school I passed every day before they came to us.

Despite the conditions of my childhood, I was lucky to have wonderful and loving parents who taught us the simple truth about love and respect for all humankind. It was strange because I felt they had so much to be resentful of. But my parents worked hard and hoped and prayed for a better world for their children. What my parents taught me I came to understand later in life as the philosophy and discipline of nonviolence and love. In 1955, when I was fifteen years old, I went to Montgomery, Alabama—just fifty miles from my home—and heard for the first time Dr. Martin Luther King, Jr., talk and preach about nonviolent protest. Dr. King's words inspired me. He dared to stand up to an oppressive system. He stood with Rosa Parks and 50,000 others who one day in 1955 said "no more." For the 381 days of the Montgomery bus boycott, courageous men and women chose to walk in dignity rather than ride in humiliation in the back of the bus. So I burned with the desire to know more about nonviolent, peaceful protest. I immersed myself in the philosophy and learned at an early age that America was deeply divided over race. I also learned that America was profoundly ready for a lasting peace—a bridge of reconciliation between the two worlds, one black and the other white.

During the 1950s and 1960s, America could not ignore the clarion call for racial reconciliation. Dr. King once said, "If we fail to live together as brothers and sisters, we will perish as fools." For him—for all of us, really—the choice was, and is, between reconciliation and nonexistence. During the 1960s, I saw civil rights workers and courageous people in towns and cities throughout the South fighting to tear down the tyranny of segregation. I saw them with their heads cracked open by nightsticks. I saw them in Selma, in Montgomery, in Birmingham, lying in the streets, weeping from tear gas, calling helplessly for medical aid.

I saw a woman and young children who were marching in peaceful protest run down by policemen on horses, beaten by fire hoses, and chased by police dogs. Yet these people were warriors in a moral revolution, a revolution of values, a revolution of ideas. They wanted to redeem the very soul of America. Our struggle was not a physical struggle against coldhearted authority but a moral struggle for the hearts and souls of our fellow human beings.

Our struggle meant that we had to embrace the philosophy and techniques of nonviolence as a means for social change. When we marched across the Edmund Pettus Bridge in Selma in 1965, we were saying through our civil disobedience of unjust laws that we had faith in higher principles. Our hearts were full of forgiveness. Our minds knew the meaning of acceptance, and we were guided by the spirit of reconciliation.

Today, I believe with all my heart and soul that means and ends are inseparable. If our goal is a beloved community of peace, love, and justice, then our tactics cannot include war, hate, and bitterness against those who jailed us, beat us, and even killed us. When we suffered violence and abuse, our concern was not for retaliation. We sought to understand the human condition of our attackers and to accept our suffering in the right spirit. When nonviolence was for some merely a tactic for social change, for many of us nonviolence became a philosophy, a way of life, a way of living.

During the past forty years, I have traveled the length and breadth of our country and met people from all walks of life. People often asked me, "Don't you despise those men who beat you and jailed you over forty times?" My answer may surprise you: I have no malice toward them. Hate is too heavy a burden to bear. Hatred and revenge will destroy both you and me. It will eat away at your very soul, your very essence. If you let hate and revenge control you, you cannot build the beloved community—you cannot build one house, one family, one nation if you are not somehow consumed by the spirit of love and reconciliation.

Some have asked me how I could possibly forgive George Wallace and Bull Connor. This is, in part, how: I see those who defended segregation as victims of history, tradition, and custom. In a sense, we are all victims of our circumstances until we have that moment of clarity when we recognize the dignity and worth of all human beings. You may despise the ways and actions of a person, but you might not despise him. He may deliberately try to harm you, but you still have to love him until he loves himself.

In the 1950s, we experienced a U-turn in American history sparked by the demand for justice that opened new paths in our journey toward a truly democratic society. When I was twenty-four, as chairman of the Student Nonviolent Coordinating Committee I traveled to the state of Mississippi to help organize the Mississippi freedom summer. I went to Mississippi because of the systematic oppression of poor blacks in the Mississippi delta. In 1964, it was almost impossible for most people of color living in the old states of the confederacy to register to vote. As a result, the state of Mississippi had a black voting-age population of more 450,000, but only about 18,000 were registered to vote. In Lowndes County, Alabama—located between Selma and Montgomery—80 percent of the residents were African American, but there was not one single African American registered to vote.

We began organizing in Mississippi with one simple mission: to register as many black voters as possible. I will never forget that summer. Students, teachers, lawyers, doctors, ministers, priests, rabbis, and nuns arrived from all over the country to work in freedom schools, where black citizens were taught how to pass the so-called literacy test. They came to help register people to vote, to open up the democratic process. There was a spirit of excitement, a spirit of love for America's promise. Those who came to Mississippi cared deeply for America, and no force could turn them away. Yet freedom did not come without a heavy cost. Less than a month after we arrived, three civil rights workers, young men that I knew—Andy Goodman, Mickey Schwerner, and James Chaney—disappeared. We did not know what to think; we hoped for the best, but feared the worst. Two days later, the car of these three young workers was found buried in a swamp. It was more than six weeks before their bodies were discovered. These three young men had been arrested, taken to jail, turned over to the Klan, then beaten, shot, and killed. These three young men did not die in Vietnam; they did not die in the Middle East; they did not die in Africa. They did not die in Eastern Europe, or in Central or South America. They died in our own country for the right of all of our citizens to become participants in the democratic process.

I tell this story because we knew that our cause was just and right; it could never be subdued by a bullet, a fire hose, or the murder of a fellow civil rights worker. But those of us in the movement learned in that time that our struggle was not for a month, a season, or a year. We learned that it is the struggle of a lifetime. That is what it takes to build the beloved community.

To succeed, we must dedicate ourselves to reconciliation every hour of every day of every week of every year. The movement instilled in many of us the dream that we could—through disciplined nonviolent action—transform this nation into the beloved community. This was our conscious goal. We knew we had to possess a faith in humanity, a willingness to believe that we have the moral capacity and ability to care for one another. When, as a young student, I sat down at a lunch counter in Nashville, I did not fear for my life. Somehow our desire for justice was greater than our instinct for survival. We had been trained in nonviolent protest: if attacked, we would not resist. We were taught to suffer and find redemption in passive resistance to force. The Nashville police had weapons, the law, and southern customs behind them. All we had was the conviction that those laws and customs were not right. We sat at the lunch counters as mobs attacked us, taunted us, and spit in our hair. I was arrested that day for the first time, along with others. We had been sitting in an orderly, peaceful, nonviolent fashion, yet the charge against us was disorderly conduct. And even though I was arrested, I felt no shame or disgrace. Nor did I feel fear. As we were led out of the store singing "We shall overcome," I felt deep joy, elated and protected by a power greater than me.

I had been told by my mother, my father, my grandparents, and my great-grandparents, "Don't get in trouble!" But I got in trouble—it was good trouble. It was necessary trouble. It felt holy, and noble, and good. That day my peaceful protest unlocked the door to racial reconciliation. I could not win by being like they were—fearful of change, hateful, and suspicious. I had to demonstrate who we could be—loving, trusting, and committed to a higher idea of human relationships. I think my personal journey of reconciliation began in that moment. I understood then, as I do now, that reconciliation begins with forgiveness. It calls upon us to love and not to hate, to heal and not to kill, to build and not to tear down.

Our nation's need for reconciliation extends beyond our struggle for civil rights in the twentieth century. We have forced Native Americans from their land, we have imprisoned Japanese Americans, we have used fear and suspicion to defend actions that were wrong. And we have systematically denied opportunity to our own people because of their race, their religion, their sex, their sexual orientation, or their ethnic background. For a great nation such as ours, it is very difficult for us to admit our mistakes. But reconciliation requires no less.

My great-grandparents were slaves. They labored on plantations and were never paid for their days upon days of back-breaking work. When I look at the institution of American slavery, I believe we are ready in our hearts for an official apology by the Unites States government. Our government has never apologized, nor issued a formal apology on behalf of the American people. This one simple act would speak volumes about who we are as a nation and a people. This is not an issue of black and white, but of right and wrong. As a black man, I do not blame any white person for slavery. The responsibility for slavery rests with a nation, a government, and a culture that allowed this cruel, inhumane system to exist. We do not seek an apology to assign blame, but to acknowledge a great wrong. There is a lot of pain flowing from the blood of the battlefields of Gettysburg and Appomattox. Many decades later, there is still a lot of hurt from this dreadful, inhumane, and divisive institution. We need to get it out. Though 150 years have passed, slavery has a deep connection to our race problems today. We need to set the truth free. We need to put our cards on the table face up. By doing this, we can speed our nation's journey toward reconciliation.

For more than forty years, I've made it my business, my life's work, to help tear down the walls that separate us and to build in their place bridges of reconciliation. Several years ago, I felt that the members of Congress needed to examine race relations in their communities. To my surprise, many members did not know where to begin racial dialogues in their own communities. So I started to organize congressional dialogues on race with a colleague from New York—Amo Houghton, a Republican. As part of the dialogue, Congressman Houghton and I led our first Civil Rights Pilgrimage to Birmingham, Montgomery, and Selma in 1998. We've made this pilgrimage every year since then. In a sense, these annual pilgrimages could be called journeys of reconciliation, journeys to uncover the philosophy of nonviolence and discover the stories of those who were true American patriots, defenders of justice and freedom in the 1950s and 1960s.

On these journeys we bring together members of Congress, their families, and staff members, and we travel to the deep South. Many of our participants have never been to the South. We travel the path of the movement, singing freedom songs and listening to testimonies from my colleagues in the movement. Several members have broken down and cried on their visit to the 16th Street Baptist Church in Birmingham, where four little girls were killed in 1963. The pilgrimage usually either ends or begins with a walk across the Pettus Bridge in Selma to commemorate the anniversary of the march from Selma to Montgomery. This is a powerful symbolic moment for everyone. I tell them the story of how state troopers beat us and tear-gassed us in 1965. But now, as we walk across the bridge, we are greeted by state troopers who include women and minorities among their numbers. In 1965 there was not a single woman, not a single African American or Hispanic or Asian American in those ranks. When I went there last year with my wife Lillian, with President Clinton leading the group, the state troopers —white and black, men and women—saluted us. And on the other side of the bridge, the governor of Alabama met us and said to me, "Welcome home!" Some may call this a symbolic gesture, but I believe it says something about laying down the burden of race and creating a sense of community with a heart of forgiveness, a mind of acceptance, and a spirit of reconciliation. There is power in symbols, and in symbolic actions.

We cannot afford more war. We cannot risk hurting our fellow human beings with hatred and suspicion and mistrust. We instead have to love others as we love ourselves. We are told in the Bible that humankind should beat their swords into ploughshares, their spears into pruning hooks, neither shall they study war anymore. The forces of division may destroy one person, but the idea of peace and reconciliation will build a new world order. This will be a world not polarized or separated or locked in struggle, but a beloved community, truly at peace with itself and reconciled.

The bridge of reconciliation will not be built overnight. It is not an easy task. In fact, it is the most difficult human endeavor I can imagine. It is harder than going to the moon, or exploring the depths of the sea. The bridge of reconciliation requires us to us reorder our way of thinking, being, and behaving.

We must help one another. We have an obligation to help one another through life—by working for each other, by pushing for each other, and by pulling for each other. The world today is a different world than the one in which I came of age during the 1960s. We are fortunate that the visible signs of racial injustice are gone; but the scars and stains of racism, separation, and division still remain. In our hearts we know that there is still work to be done before we are truly reconciled, before we can build a beloved community. So I say to each and every one of us: whatever it is that you care about—better health care, education, the environment, working conditions, civil and human rights—pick your cause and make your contribution. We have an obligation, a mission, and a mandate to do our part in building the beloved community, in building bridges of reconciliation.

I close with a story. When I was growing up outside of Troy, Alabama, fifty miles from Montgomery, I had an aunt by the name of Seneva. My Aunt Seneva lived in what we call a shotgun house. I know that many of my readers today don't know what a shotgun house is. It is an old house with a tin roof where you can bounce a ball (to use a nonviolent image) through the front door and the ball will go straight out the back door. In a military sense, a shotgun house is an old house where you can fire a gun through the front door and the bullet will go straight out the back door without hitting anything. My Aunt Seneva lived in such a house. She did not have a green manicured lawn; she had a simple dirt yard. From time to time she would walk out into the woods and take branches from a dogwood tree and make a broom that she would use to keep that yard very clean. In this old shotgun house, you could look up through the ceiling at night, through the tin roof, and count the stars. Whenever it rained, Aunt Seneva had to get a bucket to catch the rainwater leaking through the roof.

One Saturday afternoon, a group of my sisters and brothers and a few of my cousins and I were playing in the dirt yard and an unbelievable storm came up. The wind started blowing, the thunder started rolling, the lightning started flashing, and the rain started beating on the tin roof of this old shotgun house. My aunt became terrified. She started crying as she got us all inside the house. She thought the old house was going to blow away. She asked all us little children to hold hands, and then we started crying, too. The wind continued to blow, the thunder continued to roll, the lightning continued to flash. And when one corner of the house appeared to be lifting from its foundation, she had us walk to that corner of the house, holding hands, to try to hold it down with our little bodies. When another corner appeared to be lifting, she had us walk to that corner and try to hold the house down with our little bodies. We were little children walking with the wind. But we never left the house.

America, we must never leave the house. Our foremothers and forefathers may have come to this great country in different ships, but we are all in the same boat now. So we have to create one house, one family—the American house, the American family, the world house, the world family. We must never give up, or give in, or give out. We must continue to walk with the wind and let the spirit of reconciliation be our guide.

Toward a Vision of Reconciliation

Moving Beyond a Black/White "Race" Paradigm

Johnnetta B. Cole

We human beings continue to point out and exaggerate our differences in order to disrespect, discriminate against, and oppress each other. What will it take for us to cease to do so? How can we create and carry out a process of change that might one day turn Dr. Martin Luther King's dream into a reality? Just imagine our community, our nation, and our world as places where each and every one of us is judged by the content of our character rather than the color of our skin, the shape of our bodies, the funds in our pockets, the rhythm of our accents, and the gender of the person with whom we couple. What an exquisite, moving, powerful possibility: that we might one day come to see the content of each other's character as what matters, not how we worship a god, if we do; how young or old we are; and how we are differently able. This essay is one response to the questions of how we get to such a place—questions that will be easily dismissed by some as hopelessly idealistic, but lifted up by others of us who insist that the way things are among us, the diverse peoples of the world, is not the way they should or must be.

Moving Beyond the Black/White "Race" Paradigm

More than a century ago, the African American scholar and activist W.E.B. Du Bois prophetically observed, "the problem of the twentieth century is the problem of the color line."[1] Today, Dr. Du Bois might modify his observation to suggest that the problem of the twenty-first century is not just color, but difference—difference and the multiple ways in which systems of inequality are constructed in response to human diversity. The literature on intergroup conflicts based on our differences is vast, especially literature on the divide between what are called the black and white "races" in the United States.[2]

The black/white paradigm of "race" relations has occupied our national imagination and fueled social movements for and against it since the founding of our country. This is a legacy we will not easily put behind us. While fully acknowledging the countless expressions of white supremacy that take the form of institutionalized and individual racism directed toward African Americans, I want to move beyond this black/white paradigm to explore some crucially related issues. Before doing so, I must be very clear that I am not at all suggesting that we know everything we need to know about the black/white divide. And I am certainly not suggesting that we have discovered the key to ending racism. I am suggesting that by focusing our attention in a slightly different way—changing the angle of the lens, if you will—we might gain new and significant insights into the old "race" problem. We anthropologists are fond of saying that it is scarcely the fish that discovers water. By turning our gaze toward other and less studied issues, we sometimes gain insight into the very things that are closer and more familiar to us.

In Atlanta, where I served as president of Spelman College and later taught at Emory University, so much of our attention to "race" relations centers on the black/white paradigm, as if there are no other people of color in the city. The reality is that while African Americans are the largest group among communities of color (28 percent of metropolitan Atlanta's 3.8 million people), we will make serious mistakes if we continue to act as if Asian Americans, who are 2.8 percent of Atlanta's population, and Hispanics, who are 3.5 percent, do not exist. Clearly these communities exist and are growing. The same point can be made about university communities across the country: populations that we have not paid much attention to are becoming an important part of the student body.

Here, let me hint at the complexities of racial and ethnic relations involving a large and diverse group of people in the United States who are lumped under the single category of "Hispanics." While there are clear class, national origin, and even language differences among the many Hispanic groups in the United States, Anglo racism asserts that "those people" are all the same, whether they come from Puerto Rico,

Mexico, El Salvador, Nicaragua, Chile, Cuba, the Dominican Republic, or any of the other areas that constitute Hispanic America. And the tenacious stereotypes are destructive as well as inaccurate: "They are all lazy and looking for a handout, they all need to learn how to speak good English, and you know they are all in our country illegally."

While those of us in higher education should immediately recognize and reject such stereotypes, we should not turn away from valid generalizations about Hispanic or Latino people in the United States. When compared with white America as a whole, Hispanic people as a whole have lower incomes; are more often unemployed, underemployed, or only seasonally employed; have less access to health care and adequate housing; and are subject to all the consequences of high dropout rates from schools—many of which do not offer a curriculum that is in any way bicultural.

Any effort to understand Hispanic peoples in the United States requires that we note that there are many ways in which various Hispanic or Latino people interact and cooperate, and that there are also visible— and at times very intense—conflicts within and between these various communities.

To continue exploring issues beyond the black/white paradigm in American "race" relations, let us look at conflicts within communities of color, and then briefly raise the question of tensions and conflicts between communities of color.

Intergroup Conflicts in Communities of Color: Airing Our "Dirty Laundry" in Public

It has always been true of black folks in North America that we come in a range of colors and occupy a range of positions in American society. This is obviously a reflection of the fact that the 40 million black folks here in the United States are a people with a shared history, or certainly a shared historical memory, who, for reasons of education, gender, sexual preference, social class, and other differences, have varying and sometimes conflicting views on any given matter.

In 1970, Vera M. Green, a distinguished black anthropologist, observed, "the stage is being set for a confrontation of diversity among persons of African descent within the United States."[3] That moment has arrived, and indeed there is no shortage of examples of difficult dialogues and even open conflict among black people from Africa, the

Caribbean, and those of us born here in the United States. Green made an important contribution in demonstrating that diversity among black folks in America was not new, and that the "descendants of Africans in the United States" had always been culturally varied. Moreover, she asserted that research by black scholars paid attention to such diversity while studies by white scholars tended to ignore it.[4]

But when we speak of "the black community," how often we immediately conjure up images of a desolate urban landscape filled with poor people who are failing miserably. And, as recent debates about intelligence and race illustrate, the myth that there are genetic bases for differences in the intelligence of black and white people persists despite overwhelming evidence to the contrary.[5]

My point is that, in trying to explain intergroup differences—such as differences between black and white students—the tendency is to represent each group as internally homogeneous. Thus, all white people are represented as achievers and all black people are represented as underachievers. Of course, neither representation holds true when you look carefully at the people being generalized about; in any community there is a spectrum of high achievers, those who fail to achieve, and those in between. Moreover, sufficient data exists to demonstrate that, when given equal opportunities, individuals within various groups can and do excel. Thus, to understand the complexities of the black/white "race" paradigm, we must acknowledge that there are many voices within the African American and Euro-American communities of our nation, just as there are within Asian, Hispanic, and Native American groups. When we focus on the black/white divide, we erase differences within each side of that equation.

If we are to engage in genuine reconciliation around racism in the United States, it is necessary (but, obviously, not sufficient) for those of us in the diverse communities of black folks in our nation to analyze and organize against the multiple ways in which white skin privilege exists and is perpetuated through institutions and through individual behaviors. But we must also understand and struggle against the ways in which factors within our communities contribute to dangerous and destructive social patterns. There is a sense in which white racism feeds on and then is fed by certain conditions within African American communities. For example, black-on-black violence has become so pervasive that, in the words of James W. Clarke, "it is taking an extraordinary toll on young lives in America's inner cities."[6] The fact that police often turn their eyes from such incidents clearly plays a role in the continuation of—and, indeed, the increase in—such crime.

Of course, intra-group conflict and violence is not confined to black Americans. In a recent National Public Radio commentary, a young Chinese American man spoke of his years of learning to assimilate, and described being confronted one day by a group of recent immigrants from China. Their encounter ended in a fight in which one of the new arrivals asked, "Why are you fighting us? We are all Chinese." The young man's response was "No, we are not the same." Since that encounter, the commentator said, he has been on a quest to figure out how much he lost of his own cultural identity in the process of assimilation. And he continues to ask what he truly has in common with all other Chinese people, especially those raised in Taiwan or Hong Kong. To the complexities this young man was addressing, we can add the reality that, while Asian Americans experience the consequences of myths that range from "model minority" to "yellow menace," there are profound points of difference as well as similarity among Chinese, Japanese, Korean, Laotian, Cambodian, Indian, Pakistani, Vietnamese, and other peoples of Asia living in the United States.

Furthermore, intra-group tensions and conflicts not only occur within racial and ethnic communities, but also abound in other groups. For example, there are conflicts between gay men and lesbian women, and lesbian partner battering has become a critical emerging issue in the research on and advocacy against domestic violence.

As historian Dan Carter points out in his contribution to this volume, social class is a profoundly divisive force within as well as across groups, and it is one of the most significant ways by which people who share ancestry, history, national identity, and culture can be divided. In short, I am referring to the great divide between the numbers of white Americans who have and the people of color who have not, and the growing divide between the haves and have-nots within a given community of color.

Class, as represented by status—by access to resources and by consumption patterns—is a line being drawn in indelible marks across the face of black America. Unlike in the past, when black professionals often resided in the same community and even on the same block with black working-class families, today, as a result of desegregation and civil rights, middle-class African Americans may choose to live in areas where the values and property holdings definitively reflect their class. Like white folks who flee urban decline, middle-class blacks also seek refuge in suburbia. As a result, these African Americans have little contact with poor and working-class members of their "racial" group, except under circumstances where power differentials are magnified, such as in the relationships of supervisor/subordinate or employer/employee.

No longer can we assume that the person recoiling from an inner-city street kid will be white, for he or she is just as likely to be African American. And despite phenotypic similarities, the fear is real, the recoil is quick, and the satisfaction that comes with saying "I am not at all like him" is a heady perfume in contemporary American status politics. Similar examples can be found in other parts of our hemisphere and throughout the world—in any place where there are individuals who share language and some elements of culture but who are sharply distinguished by class. An indigenous Brazilian, for example, has little in common with an urbane São Pauloan. Among individuals who share national identity, geography, and language, class can create an extraordinary chasm. What else could account for the murders of Brazilian street youth that have escalated over the last decade? Confronted with embodied poverty, the police, as upholders of middle-class respectability, conspire with citizens to "eradicate" what they consider to be an impoverished blight. This "blight" is homeless children!

Issues of class difference are, of course, intimately entangled with expressions of particular values. A vivid example of value conflicts within a "racial" group can be seen in the tensions between black youth who want to "set it off"—that is, expose and explode the hypocrisy of the American dream—and working-class black families who struggle to achieve a modicum of what that dream represents in terms of a steady job and home ownership. There is tension between both groups and upper-middle-class people who, in terms of material goods and consumption patterns, have little in common. We see value turf wars writ large when African American youth linger in neighborhoods in which working-class residents harbor resentment that their streets are not safe and their homes are unprotected from this encroaching force. Ironically, black homeowners or community residents frequently do not feel comfortable calling the police, for regardless of the "race" of any particular law enforcement individual, the system itself is viewed as belonging to and operating in the interests of white people.

In this landscape of value conflict, those in the black upper-middle class rarely venture into poor black communities, and in some ways they become more aligned with white people of the same social class rather than with members of their "racial" community. This alienation means that upper-middle-class black folks will fail to play a role in community-building—a measure that could change some of the very social conditions that perpetuate the twin evils of racism and poverty.

Intergroup Conflict Among Communities of Color: "The Hate That Dare Not Speak Its Name"

If we are ever to reconcile the range of our diverse racial and ethnic differences, we must address conflicts that occur between so-called minority groups. Among the most visible of such conflicts are those between African Americans and Koreans in Los Angeles, Haitians and Cubans in Miami, and Puerto Ricans and Dominicans in New York. Such conflicts emanate from economic competition, ethnocentrism, and lack of cultural understanding. James M. Jones calls this the "new American dilemma."[7] He argues that the "old" American dilemma "arose in an era of overt racial segregation and egregious denial of basic civil and human rights" and was rooted in a paradigm of interracial conflict dominated by the two-dimensional, black/white model.[8] The new American dilemma is "set in a context of multiracial contact" and considers diverse sources of conflict between and among groups.[9]

The writer Ying Ma calls such enmity "the hate that dare not speak its name."[10] A Chinese immigrant who grew up in a black community, she speaks of the pain she encountered growing up and learning a new culture. The perpetrators of this pain were not whites, but rather poor minority (black) children like her. In a recent article in a British newspaper, we read of Asians and Caribbeans waging a bloody war. Author Darcus Howe describes a situation that mirrors the harassment Ying Ma experiences. In Britain, Asians are the perpetrators of violence against blacks. Howe describes this murderous conflict: "I mentioned that relations between Asians and blacks in Bradford were at a rather low ebb. In fact, it is much worse than that. There is much blood on the carpet. A group of Asians executed a black man, shot him and slung his body in a river."[11]

We are horrified by these acts. How, then, do we stop such violence? Certainly honesty is the first step. We must acknowledge that conflicts between communities of color exist. After this first step we can move toward greater cooperation among the very groups that can then wage more effective actions against the larger oppressive forces: white hegemony and racism.

Another essential step is quite simply the kind of broad-based education that chips away at the ignorance of one community of color about another. This kind of educational process is going on in some places through organizations like the Black-Korean Alliance in Los Angeles. In January of 2001, I attended a Rainbow Push conference that was a moving example of cooperation among people of different "racial," ethnic, gender, sexual, religious, age, and even political groups. On a personal note, I learned and grew so much from being part of a group of six black and six Jewish women in Atlanta. James Jones, writing about what he calls the new American dilemma of "race," sees the work of such organizations and groups as "promoting a bond among diverse people and enhancing joint outcomes."[12]

Surely any constructive effort to engage in the long, complex, and overdue process of racial and ethnic reconciliation—whether on our campus, in our nation, or in our world—must involve an analysis of how class structures are constituted, how political power is amassed and asserted, and how social concepts about "race" have worked to privilege one group over another. Today, as in the past, much of our analysis has centered on what I call the black/white paradigm and the intense difficulty in eliminating white racism. Though this is an awesome task in itself, as I have suggested in this essay, there are other analyses in which we must engage. Reconciling "race" relations in the United States must also involve a consideration of the multiple communities that constitute our nation as a consequence of movements and processes that we describe with such terms as immigration, borderlands, globalization, and transnationalism. And while we must continue, with increased attentiveness, to analyze the many ways in which white hegemony is expressed in the hatred of, discrimination against, and oppression of people of color, we must also lift up for analysis conflicts within communities of color as well as those between such communities.

We must also agree that while an analysis of "racial" and ethnic conflicts is a necessary beginning for a process of reconciliation to take place, it is not enough. It is far from enough. In my view, analysis must be accompanied by a belief that change is possible, and by a commitment to engage in the kinds of action that will bring about that change.

Before the civil rights movement of the 1960s, it was difficult to believe—but those of us who love freedom had to believe—that the deeply entrenched laws and practices of the American Jim Crow era would be dismantled. The destruction of apartheid in South Africa was hardly predicted a decade or so ago—except, of course, in the hearts and minds and actions of the women and men who were freedom fighters in that country. I take comfort in the words of the anthropologist Margaret Mead, who once said, "Never doubt that a small group of committed citizens can change the world. Indeed, it is the only thing that ever has."[13]

Believing that change is possible carries with it the awesome responsibility to become an agent of that very change. How do we do that? In my view, we do it by trying again and again the fundamental strategies and methods that are the backbone of the civil rights movement: voting, lobbying, and that essential human activity called educating people. In short, the ultimate reconciliation of racial and ethnic conflicts requires that we legislate, educate, and even agitate, when that is the appropriate response to discrimination and oppression. I am speaking of very basic but powerful actions:

- We must vote into office women and men who will lead us in the struggle against intolerance and all forms of discrimination.
- We must pressure our federal, state, and local legislative bodies to pass and then enforce the laws we need for full civil rights for all of us.
- We must bring into every classroom, appropriate to the subject matter being taught, the truths about human diversity and about the destructiveness of racial, ethnic, and other kinds of divisiveness.
- On university campuses, we must call out a friend who uses a racist or sexist slur, even if no people of color or women are present. We must ask classmates or colleagues what evidence they have when comments are made about all Jews, or all Arabs, about homosexuals or people who are differently abled.
- When it is time to use the nonviolent methods associated with Rosa Parks, Dr. Martin Luther King, Jr., Congressman John Lewis, and Fannie Lou Hamer—indeed, with all of the leaders of the civil rights movement—let us do so.

The goal of the precious and difficult process we call reconciliation is simply and powerfully captured for me in an American Indian expression. We strive toward a day when, in the words of the Sioux, "With all beings and all things we shall be relatives."[14]

Notes

1. W.E. Burghardt Du Bois, "The Freedmen's Bureau," *The Atlantic Monthly*, March 1901, 354.

2. I stand with those anthropologists who do not find biological evidence for something that we call a "race," although it is clear that we humans have constructed this concept and built a system of inequality called racism on the basis of that construction. Rather than taking on that issue here, I will simply put "race" within quotation marks.

3. Vera M. Green, "The Confrontation of Diversity Within the Black Community," *Human Organization* 29(4) (Winter 1970), 267.

4. Ibid., 268.

5. In October 2000, the *Wheel*, Emory's student newspaper, ran an editorial essay by a student who claimed that scientists have shown differences of intelligence can be based on race. His essay inspired not only written responses from faculty, administrators (including the president of the university), and students, but also gave voice to the anxiety that "race" was a problem at Emory, and one that the university had not dealt with in a sufficiently self-conscious way.

6. James W. Clarke, "Black-on-Black Violence," *Society*, July/August 1996, 48.

7. James M. Jones, "Psychological Knowledge and the New American Dilemma of Race," *Journal of Social Issues* 54(4) (1998), 641–662.

8. Ibid., 642.

9. Ibid., 645.

10. Ying Ma, "Black Racism: The Hate That Dare Not Speak Its Name," *The American Enterprise* 9(6) (November/December 1998), 54–56.

11. Darcus Howe, "Where Asians and Caribbeans Now Wage Bloody War," *New Statesman*, September 4, 2000, 20.

12. James M. Jones, 658.

13. "The Speaker's Electronic Reference Collection," Aapex Software, 1994. This quotation has become so well known that it is difficult to trace to its original source.

14. Black Elk, "*Hunkapi*: The Making of Relatives," in *The Sacred Pipe: Black Elk's Account of the Seven Rites of the Oglala Sioux*, recorded and edited by Joseph Epes Brown (Norman: University of Oklahoma Press), 105.

Race, Class, and Reconciliation

Dan Carter

As a historian, I am all too aware that we are constrained by our past and by the culture in which we live. If some gloomy sociobiologists are correct, our conduct is also shaped by a genetic code that echoes fictional Wall Street financier Gordon Gecko's infamous assertion: "Greed is good." But I do not believe that we are helpless prisoners of our past, our culture, or our genes. It seems to me that what makes us human is our rebellion against those very constraints and our desire to create a world that is *not* shaped alone by instinct and self-interest. Nor do I believe that true reconciliation can come if we cease to work toward these goals. I say this not as a distanced and morally neutral scholar, but as someone who is committed to the belief that we can tame, even if we cannot eliminate, the historic divisions that have separated us from each other as a people.

We have to begin by recognizing that our multiethnic and multicultural history seems to exacerbate our tendency to carve out a place in which we can insulate ourselves from those we conclude are "different." And too often that difference becomes (in our minds) a mark of superiority or inferiority. As a historian, I have come to conclude that the most divisive fault lines revolve around issues of race, class, and gender. I cannot speak to all three issues (though I think they are interrelated). Instead, my remarks are restricted to the troublesome issues of race and class in our culture.

People of color have had to deal directly with claims of white supremacy for all of this nation's history; they could not avoid it. For white Americans, and particularly those outside the South, however, it has been a sometime thing. The revolutionary generation struggled with the contradictions of a new nation that accepted human bondage even as it declared that "all men are created equal." A fratricidal civil war that grew out of the conflict over slavery forced all Americans to confront the troublesome divisions of race during the 1860s and 1870s, and nearly a century later the civil rights uprising of the 1950s and 1960s once again placed the issue at center stage.

There has always come a time, however, when whites tired of this subject. It was simply too uncomfortable to face up to our history. First there was slavery, followed by the struggle of white Southerners to maintain a separate nation built upon that institution. In the wake of emancipation and black manhood suffrage came the use of terrorism by the Klan and other vigilante groups in order to overthrow the legally constituted biracial governments of the postwar South. Black disfranchisement followed this counterrevolution only to be overshadowed by the horrific escalation of white-on-black terrorism through daily acts of violence—the most heinous of which involved the lynching of thousands of black men (and women). And then there was segregation, a hellish institution designed to systematically degrade black Southerners through the first sixty years of the twentieth century and legally exclude them from educational and economic opportunities within the region. Meanwhile, in the North, the law remained generally color-blind, but de facto discrimination existed at every level of society. No wonder we want to smooth over the rough and crooked places of our past, to dismiss the deep historical events of hundreds of years with an impatient "Get over it; that was a long time ago."

For most Americans, that depressing story has been relegated to the dustbin of the past. The majority of white Americans today would agree with the proposition that a society that accepts any form of hierarchy based upon so-called "racial" considerations is inconsistent with our democratic aspirations and incapable of achieving a meaningful reconciliation of its citizens. Only a handful of extremists openly accept the notion that genetic differences based upon race justify forms of discrimination. And it is certainly true that the cruder forms of apartheid are now gone. There are no "colored" waiting rooms, no legally segregated schools, no jobs that are openly set aside for white only workers. The destruction of legal forms of discrimination and the educational and economic advances of African Americans (and Hispanics) during the 1960s and 1970s are among the great achievements of our democracy. In 1960, black workers' earnings were less than two-thirds of those of whites; by 1980 they had increased to more than 80 percent, a dramatic change that has made possible a much larger black middle class in this nation.

But we make a terrible mistake if we retreat into smug satisfaction at the progress we have made and ignore the gap that remains between white Americans and black (and brown) Americans in this country. Of course, it is possible to pick and choose from the many statistical studies to find positive evidence about progress in race relations. But some discouraging evidence cannot be brushed aside.

Since the 1970s, the unemployment rate for African Americans has consistently remained nearly two and a half times that of whites, with slight improvements during economic upturns that are consistently erased by slowdowns in the economy. If we examine the gap between white and black income, we find that the greatest progress came in the 1960s and 1970s; the gap actually increased in the 1980s, and recent studies suggest that the gains of the late 1990s are being halted by the recent recession. Much has been made of the fact that poverty rates for African Americans and Hispanics declined significantly between 1997 and 2000, but no one remembers that between 1981 and 1995, the poverty rate for black and brown Americans actually *increased*. Most depressing of all, the percentage of black children who live below the poverty line, while also showing improvement in the late 1990s, is still a staggering one in three. And most of the more than 2 million children under age three who live in poverty (disproportionately black and brown) are not "welfare" children; 74 percent live in households that receive no public assistance.[1] These are the invisible poor.

Faced with the ongoing chasm between the status and well-being of whites and people of color in this country, we are left with the uncomfortable task of explanation. Why? What explains these depressing figures on poverty and income? Why do African Americans make up only 3 percent of the nation's doctors, lawyers, and engineers? (The percentage of black doctors actually declined between 1960 and 1990.) Why does educational achievement for African Americans continue to lag? Why has the proportion of African Americans behind bars increased 50 percent since 1950? Why are African Americans nearly 50 percent more likely to be uninsured than whites? (The figure for Hispanics is even worse.)

For much of the twentieth century, American liberals tended to emphasize the environmental factors that shaped anti-social behavior or economic disparities while conservatives resisted the notion that "immoral" choices and anti-social behavior flowed from economic deprivation or racial discrimination. (Many simply attributed it to genetic inferiority.) Most Americans, however, oscillated uneasily from one side to another, insisting upon individual responsibility while acknowledging the obligation of a society to make a special effort to assist those who begin life handicapped by racism as well as social, economic, and cultural disadvantages. In the last twenty years, however, the pendulum has clearly swung further and further to the right. While there are few conservatives who continue to defend the notion of genetic racial inferiority, the emphasis is overwhelmingly upon blaming those trapped in poverty for their own predicament. In historian George Frederickson's phrase, we have replaced racist explanations with theories of "cultural essentialism."[2]

In his 1995 book, *The End of Racism: Principles for a Multiracial Society*, the influential conservative writer Dinesh D'Souza included descriptions of a modern black "culture" of hedonism, violence, and social irresponsibility that seems little different from nineteenth- and early-twentieth-century stereotypes of shiftless and oversexed "darkies." But he also rejected the notion that genetic limitations doomed blacks to a life in the ghetto. In an argument that has been stated, restated, repeated, and stated again by other conservative ideologues, D'Souza insisted that black Americans were not victims of deprivation, poor education, racial discrimination, and a changing economy that no longer offered a ladder upward from working- to middle-class status. Instead, the poor—particularly the black poor—were victims of the foolish generosity of the welfare state constructed by liberals from the 1930s through the 1960s. This lavish welfare system had reinforced "deviant behavior" by protecting its recipients from the consequences of their anti-social actions. With a bracing dose of real-world competition made possible by the destruction of welfare programs, however, African Americans are now in a position to turn their back on this pathology of depravity and anti-social behavior and make a willful choice to embrace the conservative values of the dominant "white" culture.[3]

Of course, there was much to criticize about the nation's welfare system as it had evolved after the 1930s. Through the 1970s, Democrats as well as Republicans, welfare recipients as well as welfare critics, had talked about the demeaning effects of a system that discouraged independence. As every study shows, few people *want* to be on welfare. But those who spent time studying the problem (as opposed to issuing ideological pronouncements) always recognized that moving welfare recipients back into the nation's workforce required vast systemic changes in our political economy. Presidential candidate Clinton (as opposed to President Clinton) pointed out in 1992 that ending welfare was not likely to save money in the short run because it demanded significant budgetary allocations for training, child care, and health maintenance as well as improving the income level of low-wage workers through tax benefits and an increase in the minimum wage. By contrast, much of the conservative critique of "welfare" and the proposed "solution" (poorly compensated workfare; time limits for welfare assistance; limited expenditures for transitional educational, health, and child care assistance) has reflected little interest in any goal except reducing public expenditures for the poor. But that critique and that solution are now widely shared by most white Americans.

We should not be surprised. Since the 1960s, wealthy donors like Pittsburgh financier Richard Mellon Scaife, Colorado beer brewer Joseph Coors, oil man Fred Koch, Vicks heir H. Smith Richardson, Jr., former Treasury secretary William Simon, and many other individuals and groups have funded this conservative ideology—by one estimate to the tune of more than a *billion* dollars in the 1990s alone.[4] Year after year, dozens of conservative think tanks, "institutes," legal foundations, and research groups generate an avalanche of ideologically slanted misinformation on welfare and tax policy, misinformation that is dutifully spread by a resonating echo chamber of talk radio and right-wing interest groups. The result is a staggering degree of ignorance about the nature, the cost, and the impact of government expenditures, taxes, and social policy.

Much of this misinformation reinforces traditional racial assumptions. A 1994 CBS/*New York Times* poll found more than 81 percent of white Americans believed that blacks made up 50 percent or more of the poor in America; a similar percentage thought that most welfare recipients were black. African Americans, who make up 13 percent of the population, *are* more likely to be poor, but they make up only 30 percent of those Americans living below the poverty line and approximately one-third of those receiving means-tested government assistance. Even in the Aid to Families with Dependent Children (AFDC) program, only 36 percent of recipients in 1994 were African American, despite the fact that this program was almost entirely associated with black recipients in the minds of white Americans.[5] Although most conservative opponents of federal welfare programs sought to avoid explicit racial justifications for their view, the powerful association of welfare with (what many white voters believed was) a vast black urban anti-social and criminal underclass inevitably gave a boost to the notion that vast amounts of money are being spent on the undeserving (predominantly black) poor. Explicit racism may have declined in American life, but the similarities between the old-style racism and the new cultural essentialism are more important than the differences.

Benefits for the middle class are seen quite differently. As a *New York Times* analyst recently pointed out, the nation's tax code provides for over "$300 billion a year in tax breaks or incentives . . . for home mortgages, favorable treatment for contributions to retirement plans or college-savings plans, myriad benefits for small business ownership and stock investment." And more than 90 percent of these tax breaks go to families earning more than $50,000 a year.[6] The distinction is one that goes back to the Elizabethan poor laws. The poor (and particularly the poor who are different from us) deserve only a begrudging charity. "We all drink from wells we never dug; we warm ourselves by fires we never built," says the old Irish expression, but that is not how those of us who are middle- and upper-class Americans see our lives. Everything we receive, we have earned; we are "entitled" to our benefits.

The reality is inescapable: as we begin the twenty-first century, far more people of color than whites continue to live in the shadows of American life while the racial dimensions of disparities in income, education, health services, and treatment in our judiciary and penal system are ignored. At the same time—almost without note by policymakers, pundits, and educational reformers—in the critical area of primary and secondary education we are rapidly returning to de facto segregation in our public schools.[7] And the question that John Kennedy raised forty years ago remains no less relevant today: as long as "Negro Americans remain in the shadow of a full and free life," he asked six months before his death, "who among us would be content to have the color of his skin changed and stand in [their] place?"[8]

If we believe, as I do, that skin color is not a determinant of intelligence, creativity, or ability; if we believe, as I do, that the hand of history has laid a heavy burden upon people of color, we have a moral obligation to do more than murmur pieties about equal rights and equal opportunities.

This is not an easy task. It requires uncomfortable choices and considerable sacrifice. And this at a time when I suspect most of us would agree that "sacrifice" is not exactly the prevailing theme of our contemporary political culture. When lawmakers beholden to America's new wealthy entrepeneurial face the choice between building classrooms to replace trailers for our children or granting another tax cut to the top 2 percent of American taxpayers, it is no contest. It is easier to fill our political platforms with a rainbow of complexions, to join enthusiastically once a year on Martin Luther King's birthday to utter platitudes about equality. We insist that we are serious about the problems of racial discrimination, but our actions—in contrast to our words—treat the conundrums of race as though they were a vexatious but minor hangover from an older era.

It is much easier to relegate the uncomfortable shards of our past to a safe and comfortable category we call "history." Even the more recent past becomes the victim of those hustlers of our popular culture who have reshaped the complex history of the civil rights era into a slick pre-packaged series of rhetorical slogans that allow present injustices to live comfortably with historical memory. The great voice of the civil rights movement, Martin Luther King survives as a soothing icon to black and white, conservative and liberal alike. Thus, California businessman Ward Connerly launched his successful anti–affirmative action referendum drive on King's birthday with the announcement that Martin Luther King would have approved since he "personifies the quest for a color-blind society."

Forgotten is the Martin Luther King who dismissed such arguments in his *Stride Toward Freedom*: if a man "is entered at the starting line in a race three hundred years after another man," observed King, it was obvious that "the first man would have to perform some impossible feat in order to catch up with his fellow runner."[9] Forgotten is King's denunciation of American foreign policy in Vietnam, or his call for a "restructuring of the architecture of American society," a restructuring in which there had to be a "radical redistribution of economic and political power and wealth."[10] As Julian Bond put it, we don't like to remember "the critic of capitalism, or the pacifist who declared all wars evil, or the man of God who argued" that a nation that chose "guns over butter" would end up starving its people and destroying its soul.[11] The historical radicalism of King's call to struggle has been stripped away, leaving only a soothing pablum of feel-good sentiments.

There is actually a justification for promoting this kind of cultural amnesia. Historian Ernest Renan argues that every nation is a community both of shared memory and of shared forgetting. To the extent that we may become caught up in an endless cycle of fruitless recrimination, Renan may be right about the importance of forgetting. But I prefer the ancient wisdom of the Jewish tradition: only remembrance can bring redemption.

This does not mean that times have not changed, or that we should let our remembrance of a bitter past blind us to the journey we have made and the opportunities that lie ahead. Much has happened in the past half-century for the better as the harshest contours of American racism have been worn away by the persistent struggles of the civil rights movement. In the summer of 2000, I moved from Atlanta to Columbia, South Carolina, the birthplace of secession and the seedbed of the Confederacy. But my next-door neighbors were an African American couple who personify the American dream. He was the personnel director for a major international corporation based in Columbia, she a former assistant to the governor of South Carolina. My neighbor across the street was a successful young Chinese American attorney, my other next-door neighbor a Lebanese American cardiologist—a woman working in a specialty almost exclusively male just two decades ago. Three houses away was an African American neighbor who had just become the number two budget officer for the state. My newest neighbor, also an African American, is a highly regarded orthopedic surgeon. These are not simply tokens; they reflect the growing opportunities that exist for individuals who are given the chance to develop their abilities.

At the same time, the conflict between good and evil enacted on the television screens of the 1950s and 1960s seems far away. There are contemporary racial issues that reflect newer versions of that age-old struggle, yet often we deal not with unambiguous moral decisions, but with day-in day-out struggles to determine what is the best of a series of uncomfortable choices. How should we judge "ability" and promise in a way that is fair? Which discriminatory results are the consequence of purposeful racism, and which reflect happenstance or simply unquestioned institutional patterns? Was I denied this job because of the color of my skin? Or was the other candidate truly better qualified? Is it possible to achieve a redress of past injustices by fathers and mothers without penalizing sons and daughters? Each action, each word must be weighed; it is surely one of the most bitter and exhausting legacies of our past and our ongoing association of darker skin color with notions of inferiority.

One way to help understand the changing nature of our dilemmas is to recognize that racial ideas and attitudes increasingly reflect assumptions about class. In my Southern childhood the "single drop" theory of race was almost unchallenged. Black was black. We all know the once fashionable historical cliché about Brazilian race relations: that race was important, but "money whitened." Well, that wasn't really true about racial attitudes in Brazil, but there clearly was a difference between American and Latin societies.

Something like that change has been happening in America. I do not in any way mean to suggest that race has disappeared as a constant (if often unconscious) measure of judgment by most white Americans. Still, as the overt racism of an earlier generation declines, and a broader African American and Hispanic middle class emerges, the way is paved for whites (and some African Americans) to see "good blacks," "our kind of folks," as proof that we live in a society free of discrimination. It is a matter of "class," we are told, as though class, as opposed to race, were a legitimate means of separating our society into winners and losers.

The problem for me is that this amounts to a shift from a hierarchical society built upon the foundation of racism to one resting on the notion that there are vast differences in human beings that justify massive social and economic inequality. Increasingly that is seen as progress. Quite apart from the fact that I find such notions morally repugnant, I do not believe that true social reconciliation in our democratic society is possible unless we arrest the growing economic inequality between our citizens. Since 1979, overall income in the United States has increased over 55 percent. But the greatest increase, by far, has been for the wealthiest Americans. Over half the growth in after-tax income has gone to the top *one-half* percent of America's taxpayers, and the results are what one would expect.

In 1977, the bottom 20 percent of the American people received a little less than 6 percent of the nation's annual income, while the wealthiest 1 percent received some 7 percent. Today that bottom 20 percent receives 4 percent of the nation's annual income; the wealthiest 1 percent has seen its share almost double, to 13 percent. And today, the wealthiest 1 percent of Americans control over 40 percent of the nation's wealth, a maldistribution of wealth greater than at any time since the Great Depression.[12]

Now the argument, of course, is that a rising tide lifts all boats. With everyone growing richer, why should we concerned if some groups are a little wealthier than others?

Only that is not the case. In inflation-corrected dollars, the top 1 percent has seen its after-tax income increase 120 percent in the last quarter-century; the bottom 20 percent has actually suffered a decline of 12 percent in after-tax income. Thirty million Americans—more than half of them under eighteen years of age—still live below the poverty line; 42 million Americans have no health insurance. And despite the last ten years of steady economic expansion—once you exclude increased family income due to the growing number of dual wage earners—it was only during the last two and a half years of the 1990s that childhood poverty began to decline and the mid-50 percent of households in America saw a slight increase in income. So much for the assurances that a rising tide lifts all boats.[13]

This shift in the distribution of income and wealth stems from many sources: the internationalization of trade, the opening of a global labor economy, the decline of trade unions, and the displacement of semi-skilled and skilled workers through new technologies. But the evidence is inescapable that the growing gap between rich and poor has been exacerbated by deliberate government policies of the past two decades.

Despite all the talk of "tax cuts" in the 1980s, the bottom half of the population actually saw its taxes increase as escalating Social Security, Medicare, and excise levies, and increasingly regressive state and local taxes offset the marginal declines in the federal income tax rates. While the 50th to the 90th percentile received a very modest reduction in taxes, the nation's richest 1 percent of Americans saw an *annual* decrease of 15 percent in federal income tax liabilities in the decade of the 1980s.

These were policy decisions, deliberately made, not the inevitable consequences of free market forces beyond our control. The underlying philosophy seems to be: If you make the lives of the poor, the working class, and the marginal middle class more precarious and give them less money, they will be more productive and resourceful workers, returning benefits to society as a whole. And then if you give the rich and the well-to-do more money and make their already secure and prosperous lives even more secure and more prosperous, they will be more productive and resourceful in returning benefits to society as a whole. You think I engage in polemical exaggeration? How else can one describe the policies of the dominant national party whose main economic goals are to freeze the miserably low minimum wage for the poor and give a massive tax cut for the rich, then allow them to pass on their vast wealth to their sons and daughters?

I realize that I am on far shakier ground here. For the last thirty years, conservative think tanks have been pouring out an endless intellectual justification for this proposition: that there is a natural hierarchy of class and intelligence that functions equitably on the basis of social and economic competition, and any attempt to interfere with the unfettered forces of the marketplace can only lead us backward on that archaic and discredited path of socialism and social democracy. As Dinesh D'Souza concludes in his recent book on *The Virtue of Prosperity*, the "prime culprit in causing contemporary social inequality [in America] seems to be merit."[14]

Really? In 1974, the nation's corporate chief executive officers earned, on average, 34 times as much as their workers. By 1996, it was 180 times as much as their workers. By the beginning of this century, it was nearly 200 times as much. In 1990, the federal minimum wage was $3.80 an hour; had it grown as fast as executive pay during the decade, it would have reached more than $25 an hour by the year 2000. Are we to believe that the creativity, imagination, and productivity of corporate leaders has increased by *this* much over that of the men and women in their employ?[15]

I have a word for that kind of smug justification for the status quo; it's not one that I prefer to use in polite society.

To be fair, most of us—conservative, centrist, and liberal alike—are uncomfortable with the fictional character Gordon Gecko's unvarnished assertion that greed is good. And so we conceal the unpleasant realities of our current economic system with slogans about promoting individual opportunity, or using education as a means of redressing powerful imbalances of economic and educational opportunities, or creating "faith-based" programs that will somehow make those struggling to survive feel grateful for the fact that they are being paid miserable wages to perform miserable work without health care and, above all, without the security that most of us take for granted. At times I feel as though I am watching the captain of the *Titanic* solemnly hand out teaspoons to the passengers left on the sinking decks, with the cheery instructions: "Start bailing, you'll be fine." The truth is, those of us who are safe in our life rafts daily check our retirement portfolios as our hearts increasingly vibrate in harmony with the raucous Muzak of our contemporary culture: that clanging bell that daily opens and closes the New York Stock Exchange. Or at least we did until we learned the Wall Street musicians could hit a few sour notes.

So where can we begin?

First, I would argue that we must expand our vision of reconciliation beyond the issues of race, gender, ethnicity, and sexual discrimination to include a demand for broader economic and social justice as well as the freedom to speak and act freely.

Looking back on the last generation, we can see now that there has been a constant struggle for personal freedom and autonomy. Remember the 1960s and 1970s dictum—all politics is personal? While the battles still rage, I would argue that victory was won by social libertarians, Jerry Falwell and John Ashcroft notwithstanding. In the 1980s, there was a different kind of struggle: a battle for unrestrained economic freedom. To a considerable degree, that struggle was won by conservatives. But somehow in our headlong race for cultural and economic freedom, we have lost touch with an earlier dream most recently embodied in the call for what John Lewis describes as "the beloved community." We have come to accept as normal a society divided into the fabulously wealthy few, a comfortable upper-middle class, and half a nation one short step away from economic disaster, struggling to survive.

I do not believe real social reconciliation is possible based on these conditions. But recreating a sense of what might be—what *should* be— will not be easy.

For those of us who are committed to creating a more just society, we have to begin to search for ways to put aside those things that divide us. Many of us are particularly concerned about those disadvantaged by race, gender, ethnicity, social orientation, physical and mental disabilities. I am not going to make an attack on identity politics here, but I think we have a particular obligation to look long and hard at our own assumptions, to find ways in which we recognize that our own identity as—and here you name it—is important, but less so than the fact that we are all human.

I have spoken entirely of our need for reconciliation within our nation, but I would offer this proposition for consideration: that our inability to confront our deep divisions at home is inextricably interwoven with our delusions about the causes of our problems abroad. America's new national security policy outlined in the aftermath of September 11 rests squarely upon the twin foundations of unquestioned self-righteous-ness and unchallenged military power.[16] Although our new strategic policy pays lip service to international cooperation and improving the lives of those who live in developing countries, the ultimate solution to a world torn asunder, we are told, is for the United States to exercise its massive military power, preemptively and without warning if necessary, to thwart anyone we see as a threat.[17]

Instead of striving for an international order that is marked by greater justice, equity, and cooperation, we offer only the shaky promise of "progress" through the globalization of the world economies under the direction of international corporate interests. Instead of seeking to understand what drives people to commit acts of cruelty and violence, we divide ourselves into the good—the United States and those who support us—and the evil—terrorists and all who oppose us. Instead of policies aimed at addressing, however imperfectly, some of the root causes of these bitter divisions, we have only blustering promises to "rid the world of evil."[18]

Those of us who make our living writing and talking and teaching have an inordinate faith in the importance of the word, but it is true that language and the assumptions that our language reflects help to shape the choices of our society. Today we live in America, Incorporated, in which individualism operating within the framework of the corporate-ruled marketplace reigns with only a murmur of protest. Well, let me enter my dissent. As a means of creating wealth, corporate capitalism has a positive place in our culture, but increasingly we have come to see that marketplace as an impartial arbiter of social good rather than what it has always been: a politically charged free-for-all in which vested power increasingly places its heavy thumb on the scales of justice. As a society we increasingly resemble the cynic described by Oscar Wilde. We know the price of everything and the value of nothing.

I do not underestimate how hard it may be to challenge the ideological matrix of our new world, for words have been corrupted in truly Orwellian fashion. As he stood upon the scaffold, the Puritan martyr Richard Rumbold denounced with his last words the notion that "Providence had sent a few men into the world, ready booted and spurred to ride, and millions ready saddled and bridled to be ridden." But today those who are booted and spurred no longer swagger and proclaim their God-given right to exploit those beneath them; now they speak with the voice of humility and concern—everyone feels everyone's pain—and there is much talk of offering a helping hand to those in need.

Well, I propose that we all become cantankerous naysayers whose main duty is simply to remind all who will listen that those of us who are comfortably settled atop the pyramid of our unequal society are always ready to talk about "compassion." But there is another language that has come from authentic social movements bent on changing our society by breaking down the barriers that divide us: the struggle for economic justice in the 1930s; the fight for racial equality in the antislavery and civil rights movement; the ongoing demand that women be treated as equals. . . .

A few years ago, we left one century of continuous war and moved into another of ceaseless bloodshed. And well before the end of that century, we lost sight of the possibility of an America that demanded something greater from its citizens than the exercise of self-interest. Unless we are once again willing to imagine in new ways a world and a nation in which the dignity and worth of every person is more than an empty slogan, this is the world our children and our children's children will inherit. The only hope I can offer is to remind us all that authentic political movements struggling for justice have emerged when least expected. And they seldom bubble up from colleges and universities. As one of my favorite writers said, a keen sense of irony has seldom led anyone to mount the barricades. Our task in the future is not to lead, but to be a part of that struggle.

Notes

1. Andrew Hacker, *Two Nations: Black and White, Separate, Hostile, Unequal* (New York: Charles Scribner's Sons, 1992), pp. 97–99; www.jointcenter.org/DB/factsheet/chilpovt.htm. The last reliable statistical information we have on these and other critical economic issues comes from data gathered for the 2000 census at the height of the economic upturn of the 1990s. Unfortunately, it will be some time before we can fully measure the impact of the current recession as well as the impact of the welfare law change enacted in 1996, but the first signs are not encouraging. The United States Census Bureau released preliminary figures for 2001 in the fall of 2002 and, not surprisingly, they showed an increase in poverty from the 1999–2000 figures. *New York Times*, September 29, 2002, C-1.

2. "Demonizing the American Dilemma," *New York Review of Books*, October 19, 1995, p. 16. An exception would be *The Bell Curve: Intelligence and Class Structure in American Life* (New York: Free Press, 1994), in which authors Richard Herrnstein and Charles Murray continue to defend the notion that blacks are, in "cognitive" terms, genetically inferior.

3. D'Souza, *The End of Racism: Principles for a Multiracial Society* (New York: Free Press, 1995).

4. *Wall Street Journal*, October 12, 1995, p. 1; *Washington Post*, May 2, 1999, p. 1; May 3, 1999, p. 1. Haynes Johnson, *The Best of Times: America in the Clinton Years* (New York: Harcourt, 2001), pp. 260–64; Alan Crawford, *Thunder on the Right: The 'New Right' and the Politics of Resentment* (New York: Pantheon Books, 1980), pp. 3–41.

5. Martin Gilens, *Why Americans Hate Welfare: Race, Media, and the Politics of Antipoverty Policy* (Chicago: University of Chicago Press, 1999), pp. 68, 147. For a discussion of the connection between race and welfare, see Gillens and Jill Quadangno, *The Color of Welfare: How Racism Undermined the War on Poverty* (New York: Oxford University Press, 1994); Herbert J. Gans, *The War Against the Poor: The Underclass and Antipoverty Policy* (New York: Basic Books, 1995); and Michael B. Katz, *The Undeserving Poor: From the War on Poverty to the War on Welfare* (New York: Pantheon Books, 1989). Thomas and Mary Edsall described the political linkage between such racial issues and other social and economic issues in *Chain Reaction: The Impact of Race, Rights, and Taxes on American Politics* (New York: W.W. Norton, 1991).

6. *New York Times*, September 29, 2002.

7. Gary Orfield, *Schools More Separate: Consequences of a Decade of Resegregation* (Cambridge: The Civil Rights Project, Harvard University, 2001). As Orfield and his fellow researchers have shown, the racial integration of public school students reached a peak in the late 1980s, but as a consequence of continuing housing segregation patterns and an increasingly conservative federal judiciary, racial resegregation has increased steadily during the past ten years, North and South.

8. *New York Times*, June 12, 1962.

9. King, *Stride Toward Freedom: The Montgomery Story* (New York: Harper & Brothers, 1958).

10. From King's testimony before Congress in *Hearings Before the Subcommittee on Executive Reorganization of the Committee on Government Operations, United States Senate, Eighty-Ninth Congress, Second Session, December 14 and 15, 1966, Part 14* (Washington, DC: United States Government Printing Office, 1967), 2981.

11. *Seattle Times*, April 4, 1993.

12. *New York Times*, September 5, 1999, p. 14; see also Edward N. Wolff, *Top Heavy: A Study of the Increasing Inequality of Wealth in America* (New York: Twentieth Century Fund Press, 1995); Frank Levy, *The New Dollars and Dreams: American Incomes and Economic Change* (New York: Russell Sage Foundation, 1999); and Kevin Phillips's more popular (and polemical) *Wealth and Democracy: A Political History of the American Rich* (New York: Broadway Books, 2002). The most recent work (January 2003) is by Thomas Piketty and Emmanuel Saez, "Income Inequality in the United States, 1913–1988," and it shows a continuing growth in inequality and a general stagnation in the earning levels of Americans below the top 20th percentile. See www.papers.nber.org/papers/W8467.

13. Any number of economists have effectively refuted the argument that income has risen for the poor as well as for the rich. (For a particularly sardonic critique of these arguments—and the motivations of those who promote them—see Paul Krugman, "What the Public Doesn't Know Can't Hurt Us," *Washington Monthly* (October 1995), pp. 8–12. At the same time, extensive studies of social mobility show that the claim that social mobility in the United States is widespread (in contrast to other advanced industrial democracies) is a myth. See the overview of rel-

evant research by Gordon Marshall and Adam Smift in "Research: Social Mobility —*Plus ça change . . . ,*" *Prospect* (November 1995), pp. 85–87.

14. *The Virtue of Prosperity: Finding Values in an Age of Techno-Affluence* (New York: Free Press, 2000), p. 187.

15. One of the best brief surveys of this shift in income distribution and its impact upon American society was John Cassidy's 1995 article in the *New Yorker*, "Who Killed the Middle Class?" October 16, 1995, pp. 16–23.

16. "The National Security Strategy of the United States of America," released by the White House on September 22, 2002, is readily available on any number of websites; the doctrine of preemption was first introduced explicitly in President Bush's June 1, 2002, West Point graduation speech in which he argued that deterrence and containment were no longer sufficient; changed circumstances would require that Americans be ready to embrace the doctrine of "preemptive action." *New York Times*, June 2, 2002.

17. "While the United States will constantly strive to enlist the support of the international community, we will not hesitate to act alone, if necessary, to exercise our right of self defense by acting preemptively. . . ." "National Security Statement," p. 6. The notion of choosing the right to engage in preemptive war marks a dramatic shift from the basic tenets of international law and the policies of this nation as they were outlined by Supreme Court Justice Robert Jackson, the American prosecutor at the Nuremberg trials, when he argued in his opening remarks that "whatever grievances a nation may have, however objectionable it finds the status quo, aggressive [i.e., preemptive] warfare is an illegal means for settling those grievances or for altering those conditions." *Nazi Conspiracy & Aggression*, vol. 1, chap. 7 (Office of the United States Chief Counsel for Prosecution of Axis Criminality, United States Government Printing Office, Washington, 1946.)

18. The quote is from President George W. Bush's speech in the National Cathedral three days after the September 11 attack. *New York Times*, September 15, 2001.

All God's Children Got Shoes

Social Justice and Reconciliation

Joseph E. Lowery

My essay begins with a story you probably know: the story of the prodigal son, from the fifteenth chapter of Luke. But I set the story on a plantation in the South, about 150 years ago. One Sunday morning on this plantation, the slaves stood outside a church and listened to the worship service through the window. On other occasions they were permitted to sit in the back or the balcony, but for whatever reason, for this particular service these slaves were sitting outside, listening through the window. They heard the messages and the songs about brotherhood and heaven, and all those good things that we hear in churches. And after the service was over, they stood and watched the worshipers, all white, go back up the hillside to their respective places of abode, dressed in their Sunday-go-to-meeting clothes and their shiny shoes. The slaves then sat down beneath the shade of a spreading oak and organized a little ad hoc plantation theological seminary, and did exegesis on what they'd heard coming out the window of this church that Sunday morning.

The dean of the new seminary would look at the students and he'd say, "Heaven!" and the students would antiphonally cry back, "Heaven!" And then he'd say, "Everybody talking about heaven ain't going there." Later on in the discussion, barefooted as they were, they looked at each other and said, "You know, I got shoes." They looked at the shiny, beautiful shoes of the worshipers, and their own bare, bruised, shoeless feet, and they said, "Yeah, we got shoes, you got shoes, all God's children got shoes."

What they were saying was really the theological as well as pragmatic basis of the movement for social justice: all God's children got shoes. Even in the classical age, in the Greek state, when a person saw children playing in the yard he could always tell the children of the householder from the children of the slave by the fact that the children of the householder had on shoes while the children of the slave were barefoot. Shoes became a symbol of the householder. And so when the slaves said, "I got shoes," they were denying their exclusion from the household of God the Father. I don't think we can begin a journey of reconciliation without embracing the basic premise that all God's children got shoes, that all of us belong in the household of the Creator. Eleanor Roosevelt, a pioneer of human rights, once said that universal rights begin in small places—in classrooms, in the workplace, around the kitchen table. Perhaps we've depended too much on formal institutions and not enough on what happens around the kitchen table at the knees of parents, what happens beside Dad's comfortable rocker, what happens in the early years of the child's classroom. There's no gainsaying the fact that we've come a long, long way, but the truth of the matter is that that statement is incomplete; it is only finished when we note we've got a long, long way to go. Today, the unfinished tasks of social justice and human rights need to be addressed in small places, so that we can continue the journey to reconciliation.

I would argue that we are witnessing the passing not just of a century, and the passing into a new millennium, but the passing of an era. We have moved out of what I call the old anti-communist hysteria era into an era yet undefined. Those of us who have concerns and commitments in the area of social justice—commitments to the coming together of the people of this community and of this nation under God—need to seize every opportunity to have a voice in redefining this nation, this era. During the old hysteria era, we neglected democratic principles and institutions. We sacrificed ideals, trivialized social sensitivity, minimized the ethical, maximized the expedient; we glorified violence, sanitized the electric chair, demonized the saints, and canonized the devil—all in the name of fighting the evil empire. We have sown the wind, and we are reaping the whirlwind. We have abandoned the good spouse of spirituality, and we are having an affair with the prostitute of materialism and greed. It is an incestuous affair, and produces offspring with congenital defects—racism, sexism, classism, economic, political, and judicial violence, gun addiction, drug addiction, domestic and international terrorism.

Part of the power to redefine our nation lies in the universities of this country. In this transition, the voice of the coalition of conscience—those who focus on social justice and reconciliation from their various disciplines and experiences, those on campuses and in movements and in the church—must make itself heard. We must revitalize that coalition of conscience and help redefine this new era. The nation has experienced many shining and defining moments: the Boston Tea Party, Crispus Attucks and his fellows in the Revolution, the Bill of Rights, the Declaration of Human Rights, the Emancipation Proclamation, the Gettysburg Address, the 1954 Supreme Court *Brown* decision, and the Montgomery bus boycott. All these were defining moments in our history, moments when the downtrodden and oppressed said, "We've got shoes and we can use them to walk in dignity." And in all of these moments, people were working for something that Paul, in his letters to the Corinthians, called the common good. In every defining moment in our history, there is that focus on the common good that defines America at its noblest level, that embraces the principles and tenets and policies and practices that directed their efforts toward developing the common good.

If we are serious about social justice and reconciliation, we must establish a ground rule—we must get those shoes out—to make sure that everyone has economic justice. The dividing forces in our world are as much economic as they are theological, spiritual, ethical, moral, or legal. The division in our society around the issue of class is a devastating force that prevents us from coming together as a community and working for the common good. And these disparities, these gaps, are widening. Less than 20 percent of the people control more than 80 percent of the wealth. I would suggest that that is not even close to an equitable distribution of God's wealth.

Let me review my terms here for a moment. I like the term "equity" because "equality" seems to confuse folks, whereas you can explain "equity" with a dollar sign and everyone understands it. There is a distinction between equality and equity that perhaps I can demonstrate with a story. Some years ago, a farmer down in south Georgia developed a rabbit sausage because he had a lot of customers who didn't like pork. It was good sausage, and it did very well on the market—until a terrible thing happened. Rabbits became scarce. The farmer almost panicked, but he decided he would substitute horses for rabbits—there were a lot of old horses in his area, so he wouldn't run out of meat anytime soon. So he substituted horses for rabbits but decided to keep calling it rabbit sausage. At some point, the health folks came in and said, "Wait a minute, we think you are misrepresenting your product. We understand you call it rabbit sausage, but it's really horse sausage." And the farmer said, "No, sir, it's equal. I guarantee it's equal." So they asked him, "How do you make it?" "Well, I'll tell you," he said. "Every time I put in one rabbit, I put in one horse." I suggest that while one rabbit and one horse may very well be equal, it certainly isn't equitable. When we look at building a foundation for a community, we have to grapple with economic equity—not just equality—in this country.

When we organized the Southern Christian Leadership Conference in 1957, the median income of African Americans was about 57 percent of the median income of white Americans. Since that time, the median income of African Americans has risen to about 60 percent that of whites. It took us 44 years to get a 3 percent increase. We've got a tough struggle ahead of us because that economic inequity is a significant barrier to social justice. I agree with President Bush that individuals and private institutions, like churches and charities, have a moral responsibility to deal with these issues. But I think he is wrong to expect that they can pick up the slack in terms of economic justice. Private institutions and private citizens ought to help, but that does not relieve the responsibility of government to embrace public policies that contribute to the equitable distribution of opportunity and resources and wealth in this country.

President Bush is talking about charity. I am talking about love. And, like the distinction between equality and equity, there is a distinction between charity and love. Charity is a good thing, but it's selective; love is inclusive. Charity is seasonal; love is everlasting. Charity will give a hungry man a fish sandwich. Love will teach him how to fish. Love will provide job training opportunities for him, with a livable wage, so that he can buy his own fish sandwich. Love will see that he has good working conditions, and health care, and a pension program. Love checks the water he fishes in to make sure it is not polluted. Love is broader, more extensive, more powerful, more inclusive than charity. While I want to see charity, we cannot let public policy evacuate its responsibility for love because it puts upon private institutions the responsibility for charity.

So the issue of economic justice, in the service of reconciliation, demands love; and next to the issue of economic justice is criminal justice. It is impossible for us to achieve reconciliation and economic justice when our prisons are crowded with minorities, young people, and the poor. In Georgia, the corrections budget is exploding because we use prisons and punishment as the sole means of dealing with crime while we ignore the issue of prevention through love and economic justice.

When I was a pastor in Birmingham, a little boy who lived in the tenement house across the street from the church was arrested for breaking into a drugstore about four blocks away. I went to see the judge and asked him to let the boy go and take me instead, or even me and the judge instead, because we are more responsible for what happened than the boy. There were seven children in that boy's family and no father to take care of them; he had not been able to find work, so he had to leave because the welfare system would not help as long as he was around, whether he had a job or not. The little boy's sister was very sick, so that boy had gone to the drugstore, broken the window of the pharmacy, and taken an armful of medicines in a desperate attempt to save his sister. It is right to condemn stealing, but if we don't also work on systemic conditions that put people in desperate situations, we are not doing enough.

In the state of Georgia, most of our counties have no public defender system; those who do manage to get defense are working with lawyers who are appointed to their cases, who are not paid very much, and who do as little as they possibly can. As a result, most of the people in jail are there because their lawyers made deals in order to save time and effort. Social justice is precluded in a state that is blind to why the prisons are filling up; and it cannot be present in a system in which the poor go to jail and the rich go to Hilton Head. According to the Office of Criminal Justice Research in Atlanta, black drug offenders in Georgia are sent to prison at five times the rate of white drug offenders. Black males in Georgia are four times more likely to end up in prison than white males, and black females are three times more likely to go to jail than white females. If the mothers of the community are going to prison, who is taking care of the children? What does this mean for the future of the family? I would argue that it portends social chaos, not social justice. Blacks make up less than 30 percent of the Georgia population, but 70 percent of its prison population. If you think that is because blacks commit most of the crimes, you are not looking deep enough. The incarceration rate for blacks in Georgia has risen 83 percent since 1990, but during that same time crime rates have been going down. The use of cocaine is pretty much evenly distributed among blacks and whites, but in the year 2000 in Georgia, out of 4,100 offenders sent to prison for cocaine, 83 percent were black, according to the Georgia Department of Corrections.

And as we move toward the privatization of prisons, the situation will only get worse. When you're talking about incarceration for profit, there won't be any profit unless there are a whole lot of people in the prison. That is no way for a civilized, democratic, sensitive, ethical society to deal with its criminal justice system. Those of us who are members of the coalition of conscience must wrestle with this problem.

The week before the Reconciliation Symposium at Emory, we celebrated the birthday of Dr. Martin Luther King, Jr., but we sat silently by and ignored the problems in the criminal justice system, the one system that has been the least impacted by social change in Georgia. Yet if we are truly going to honor Dr. King, we need to move beyond honoring an individual. By honoring the missionary and ignoring the mission, by decorating the messenger and disregarding the message, we have done a disservice to Dr. King. He certainly deserves it more than any individual, but if we stop there, we betray the calling to social justice. It is all too possible to place Dr. King on some rotunda of sentimental irrelevancy and separate him from where we cross in the crowded ways of life. We could too easily immunize him and his message from the marketplace, which knows the price of everything but the value of nothing. When we passed legislation to make his birthday a holiday, it was not because Dr. King was a nice fellow, or even a great orator, or scholar, or preacher; it was because he represented the nation's commitment to racial justice, human dignity, and peace with justice.

One thing we must do to honor Dr. King is to recommit ourselves to the principle of affirmative action. There can be no social justice or reconciliation without compensation, without the adjustment of inequity. Affirmative action represents intentionality; the gap between whites and minorities was created through intentional acts of public policy and social practice, and it must be undone through intentional acts of public policy and social practice. If you hammer a nail into a board and then expect the nail to come out by itself, you're in trouble. If you think it will come out through prayer alone, you're in trouble. You have to turn the hammer around and use the claw, use the same intentionality to pull the nail out that you did to put it in. If two fingers on one hand are infected, you'd better give some intentionality to those two fingers. You can argue about whether that is preferential treatment if you want to, but I suggest you take care of the two fingers as quickly as you can—not just for the sake of the two fingers, but for the sake of the whole hand.

The principle, even theology, of affirmative action is this idea of doing something for the good of the whole, not just part of the whole. This principle is beautifully illustrated by the story of something that happened to a friend of mine, Harry B. Richardson, who was the first president of the Interdenominational Theological Center, and before that the chaplain at Tuskegee. Harry had to travel to Birmingham by train from a little town called Cheehaw one day. There was no station at Cheehaw, just a little waiting room—actually, two waiting rooms: one for the white passengers and a smaller one for the colored passengers. While Harry was waiting for the train, it started pouring down rain, and the roof of the colored waiting room was leaking. It was so bad that it was raining inside just as much as it was outside. Finally, Harry decided he was going to go over to the white waiting room, where it was dry, but when he looked in he saw there was a white gentleman there with his wife. The white man saw Harry, who was drenched, and said, "Sir, please come into this dry room with us. Because it's not good for me for you to be excluded." Isn't that the moral imperative inherent in affirmative action? It's not good for me for you to be excluded.

I think affirmative action is also biblically sound, because one of the parables Jesus told is about affirmative action: the parable of the good shepherd. As you'll remember from that story, the shepherd had one hundred sheep; ninety-nine of them were doing pretty well, but one of them was excluded. Ninety-nine of them had at least standard housing, adequate health insurance, some kind of dependable retirement program—those ninety-nine were doing pretty well. But one of the sheep was excluded, out there in the wilderness. And Jesus said to the good shepherd, "I won't take anything away, I don't plan to put you out. I just want you to hold fast until I return." The shepherd went into the wilderness and searched high and low, far and wide, north and south, east and west, until he found the excluded sheep and brought it into the fold. That is affirmative action, that is intentionality in closing the gap.

In our struggle for justice and reconciliation, we are on God's side. In 1982, two African American women, Maggie Boseman and Julia Wilder, were convicted of voter fraud in Pickens County in west Alabama near the Mississippi border. Their only crime was helping elderly voters learn about absentee voting and, of course, being black. At the close of their trial and conviction, we stood outside the courthouse and watched them being driven to the prison in the state patrol cars. Our heads were down, our hearts were heavy. One or two of the youths present cried, and others shouted, "Let's burn this *%*# down," referring to the courthouse. I advised them that while it would make a good fire, it wouldn't free Maggie or Julia. We went down the hill to a little church and held a brief prayer service. Following the prayers, we decided to initiate a march from Carrollton to Montgomery to free Maggie and Julia. To make a long story short, a few days before the march was scheduled, the head of the SCLC chapter in Pickens County called me in Atlanta to report the march was being attacked by the sheriff among others, and that the sheriff was discouraging black citizens from participating in the march, and giving them ham and turkeys. He advised them to stay away from "Lowery and that SCLC, because they will destroy our good relations down here." I assured him that hams and turkeys would not deter the people from standing up for justice, but when we gathered on the courthouse steps on the designated day, there were only between seventy-five and a hundred people there, when we had expected two hundred or more. "Surely black folks would not sell their souls for hams and turkeys in this age," I lamented.

We marched anyhow. It was chilly and a light rain was falling, but we were "picking them up and putting them down." And the staff said, "The cameras are here, let's spread out so it looks like there are more of us." But I said, "To heck with the camera, it's cold, let's cuddle up!" All the way there, I didn't even let my wife know how heavy my heart was. I talked to Martin, and I talked to God about this situation; I kept asking for a sign, and I kept thinking about selling the soul for hams and turkeys. When we got to Ellisville and turned the corner to go to the community center for our first stop, there were about 200 people there, with their marching shoes on and baskets with ham sandwiches and turkey sandwiches, to feed us, to work for social justice and reconciliation.

Part IV

Higher Education and
Human Rights

Practicing Reconciliation in the Classroom After September 11

Barbara Patterson

My university, like many across the country, canceled classes the day after the attack on the Twin Towers in Manhattan. During that open day, small groups of students and faculty met to mourn together, to follow the endless cascade of news reports, to talk about the issues and histories involved, and to reflect on what might be next. The following day, I met with my students in our class, "Methods of Religious Studies," reputedly the most dreaded of all courses required for the major in religious studies. Since many undergraduates lack awareness of how the choice of method shapes their understandings of religious life and meanings, the course content seems irrelevant. To engage these students, I have adopted a number of active learning strategies. While we read about the theories of methodology, we emphasize practicing specific methods using a variety of pedagogical techniques and strategies.[1] But the immense realities we faced in the wake of the first foreign terrorist attacks on American soil flattened our academic project. Religiously related behaviors and beliefs like the ones starkly before us now overwhelmed our growing knowledge of scholarly methodology. How could I respond to that day as a human, as a teacher?

Some colleagues did not address the attack at all in class and proceeded with the expected agenda, hoping to help restore a sense of normalcy. As a teacher committed to using lived experience as pedagogical tool, such a response was not possible for me. We were living a dramatic experience that was, for my discipline, highly relevant. I asked students to write about how they were feeling and what connections they might see between the events before us and the content of our class. This exercise had two goals. First, it allowed our first gathering after the tragedy to honor the immensity of what we were trying to grasp. The act of writing also provided a bridge by which we could move from numbing shock toward engagement—individually and together. Second, this exercise allowed students to be whole persons in the classroom, to feel and to think. Theories of experience-based learning and teaching assume that everyone in a learning environment brings the full repertoire of who they are, what they know, and how they know. Certainly there are brains in the classroom, but these brains are in bodies, and these bodies are from different cultures and religions. Additionally, we have different learning styles, different forms of intelligence.[2] Denying this holistic reality weakens the chances that the offered lessons will be fully received and retained.[3]

After writing while feeling and thinking for about twenty minutes, students shared what they wished to. Many wrote of their shock and grief, their fear. Many described feelings of intellectual and analytical inadequacy in the face of such a disaster; how does one make sense of such a thing? Where do we go from here? Only later did I make connections with the ideas of the conflict mediation theorist and practitioner Marc Gopen. In his book *Beyond Eden and Armageddon*, Gopen emphasizes that communities experiencing traumatic violence need time to explore, experience, express, and reflect on their grief.[4] The losses, the disorientations, the anguished needs have to be named individually and collectively. All perspectives need to be respected and heard out, even if subsequently challenged. Eventually if reconciliation is to begin, these reflections must also be shared with others beyond the community, including those who are part of the group considered to be perpetrators. Without honoring and sharing this grief, individuals and groups often stall out and never move toward healing and reconciliation that is truly transformative. Education, according to theories of experience-based pedagogy, moves or builds sequentially. Teaching and learning build from data to knowledge to analysis and synthesis.[5] Experience obviously is data, but for it to become knowledge requires more than cognitive processes. It also involves attitudinal and belief-related engagement and learning. In other words, a learning experience analyzes and constructs understanding via pragmatic, attitudinal, and behavioral as well as cognitive skills.[6] For this class to move our experience toward a transformative learning experience, we had to attend to all these outcomes for learning. Paying attention to the multiple dimensions of learning through and with this experience helped us move more deeply into our experience and discover more complex insights and conclusions.

Because the students knew that this was an experiential learning class, they were not startled by my request to write about their responses. They were used to this kind of engagement and had learned to give it the attention and time it takes in order to bear fruit. Of course, not every student publicly offered a response. Some did it later in another context in class or perhaps with another group or with me in an individual conference. But taking time that day proved to be a good decision as students built on their writing to consider more thoroughly what had happened and how they could connect the content of the class with their lives.

After this initial exercise, I divided the class into small groups and asked them to respond to the following scenario:

> You are the Religious Studies Consultant Group (RSCG) of the State Department. You have been called this morning to the White House for a meeting with the president and his staff. You are to brief them about your recommended strategies for analyzing the religious dimensions behind this attack apparently organized and implemented by the al-Qaeda movement. The president is not only looking for some initial understanding, but also wants you to propose an ongoing research protocol for determining what religious elements contribute to the decision-making processes of such religious groups. As a group of religion scholars, what is your initial response? What methods will you suggest in designing your research protocol? Name no more than three methods and defend your choices.

Their responses were wide-ranging and fascinating. Some focused their protocol using ethnographic strategies, starting with participant observation and moving toward interviews with individuals related to the movement. They hoped eventually to have access to member of al-Qaeda currently detained by Western nations. Another group also advocated using ethnographic methods but wanted to begin by interviewing Muslims in the United States who were unrelated to al-Qaeda. Other groups suggested first researching current scholarship on fundamentalist groups in Islam and interviewing the scholars who wrote these books in order to learn more about their sources. Still others chose textual analyses comparing traditional interpretations of Islamic texts with interpretations by several important imams leading the al-Qaeda movement. They hoped to analyze how certain theological positions became a political worldview that justified such levels of violence. What role did history play in these interpretations? What role did history play, period? And so it went, with the energy increasing as each student group made connections between what we had been studying and this real world event. Sure, there were naïve responses. Certainly there were incomplete ideas. But the point was to have them feel some agency making connections between their classroom learning and this shocking experience that called for a response of some kind. Hearing from each other only enriched each group's ideas of how their research response could be more thoroughly shaped.

Everyone agreed that the first remarks to the president and his staff had to emphasize that it would be inappropriate to use this one event to stereotype the majority of Muslims. They would warn against damaging overgeneralizations in the media or in any other official announcements. I could not have been more pleased by their substantive and inherently reconciliatory approach. It was learning at its best in the experience-based tradition—intellectual, holistic, analytical, and methodologically creative. When experiential learning and teaching can provide opportunities for integrative moments like this, I feel hope about the future of higher education making a pragmatic and positive difference in our lives and communities. Using this pedagogical approach, classrooms can become sites of reconciliatory teaching and learning practices.

Living and Learning Every Day in a Democracy

There are other experientially based strategies that effectively conceive, implement, and assess practices of reconciliation in any classroom. These approaches are specifically designed to take the kinds of dilemmas we were facing and will continue to face and engage them in order to connect learning to positive change in communities. Whether through simulation exercises, roles plays, group projects, reflective and structured writing assignments, field-based observation and research, lab practicums, and/or community-based research in partnership with local groups, students learn to engage ideas in order to become actively involved in shaping effective responses. The dynamic is transformative because ideas have consequences whether as a result of new research procedures and methods, problem-based solutions, reconstructed theories, or social action.

Such transformations in whatever form are at least potentially reconciliatory because teaching and learning this way privileges interconnections, webs of thinking and doing, if you will. It assumes there are important connections and insights between ideas and actions, people and practices, and problems and solutions. Teaching counts on realigning or highlighting these interconnections. This was true of experience-based teaching and learning long before the shock of 9/11. In fact, the founding philosophy of American higher education emphasized that the classroom was the crucible for the newly emerging democracy. In order for that democracy to flourish, young men and women must be prepared to relate ideas to pragmatic problem-solving responses, to reconcile differences for the common good of the new republic. In 1867, for example, President Gilman of Johns Hopkins University stated that the purpose of Hopkins was to "make less misery among the poor, less bigotry in the temple, less folly in politics, and less illness in the community." In 1908, Ralph Waldo Emerson declared that Harvard University existed in order to help students learn to serve as part of their patriotic responsibility.[7]

This American vision was revisited and updated in Ernest Boyer's 1990 book, *Scholarship Reconsidered: Priorities of the Professoriate*. Along with the Carnegie Report by the Boyer Commission on Educating Undergraduates—"Reinventing Undergraduate Education: A Blueprint for America's Research Universities" (1996)—this book asked institutions of higher education to reconsider what counted as "true" scholarship. Boyer made the case that teaching was a scholastic act. Seriously engaging even undergraduates in one's own research was a scholarly calling and production. It was to expand Boyer's understanding of teaching as a form of scholarship to include and integrate with the more traditional scholarship of research, or "discovery," as Boyer called it. Scholarship on the undergraduate level in this model asks faculty to design opportunities for their classroom teaching, as scholarship, to be a bridge to students sharing in their other forms of scholarship. Scholarship becomes a participatory act with larger purposes than the results of research. In experiential classes, the scholarship of teaching is linked with the scholarship of discovery in order to serve.

Teaching and learning that connects ideas with experience reinforces the founding leaders' hopes of shaping generations of scholar citizens. That vision has tremendous potential for reconciliatory change within our democracy and potentially with partners beyond it. Our students can be prepared people ready and able to effectively function amid the push and pull of active engagement with others for the thriving of all.[8] With adult mentoring amid engaged learning, students can well answer Hannah Arendt's plea from her book *The Human Condition*, "All I am asking is that we think what we are doing."

To intentionally shape reconciliatory classrooms, students, and teachers in our continually changing democracy and world is intellectually and experientially complex. It is always multidisciplinary, needing information and insight from every level of human knowing and doing. It can respond, therefore, to the variety of approaches and perspectives within real world situations, both local and global. But if reconciliatory teaching and learning is to happen in long-term, reciprocal, and mutually respectful relationships, academic institutions must embrace holistic teaching and learning not only inside our walls but also beyond them. We must learn to partner with communities, recognizing and learning from their knowledge while increasingly developing trust for shared action. Definitions of goals, identification of sources of problems, decisions about which intellectual issues are at stake must be engaged together. The importance of trust in these learning contexts cannot be overemphasized and highlights again the fundamentally reconciliatory dimensions of learning inherent to this approach.

It is a difficult project to live together in any setting with hopes of justice, liberty, and peace. Students and teachers have to learn how to recognize elements of a situation and negotiate for positive change. Things, categories, power dynamics, people, resources, and ideologies of a system do not remain static. There are continually new elements, new participants, unexpected demands, and emerging needs that require not only recognition but also good analysis and strong intellectual conclusions if action is to be useful and meaningful. Surely a good deal of the work of undergraduate education is to prepare students to be able to join in such processes successfully and appropriately. Opening our imaginations as teachers to consider such purposes and interactions is surely a challenge, but it is a challenge we must take up. As Parker Palmer has written in his book *To Know as We Are Known*, this is vulnerable work—even a kind of reconciliatory work in itself. Without it, learning can remain isolated from the kinds of real world needs of 9/11 and much less shocking events.

The "How" of Daily Learning Shapes the "What"

John Dewey, the renowned philosopher/activist of education from the University of Chicago, understood the need for this approach to learning as holistic and reconciliatory. The goal was strengthening communities through participation by scholar citizens. What has made the difference in reaching these goals is not so much the "what" of learning as the "how":

> "How" students learn may well have more impact on their subsequent engagement in community activities than "what" they learned. . . . [A democratic learning process] should engage students in reaching outside the walls of the school and into the surrounding community. It should focus on problems to be solved, and it should be collaborative, both among students and between students and faculty [and I would add between schools and community partners]. (Erlich 1997, 59)

If that "how" is to be reconciliatory, it must begin locally, at a specific school and in relation to a specific community. Our 9/11 class was somewhat grandiose in my choice of a presidential scenario. But the experience felt that big. More normally, experience-based teaching and learning are fundamentally place-based, meaning in a place accessible to students and teachers. Even if the eventual focus becomes broader or global, study that becomes active engagement necessarily begins where we live because it must be real enough for us to think about and collaborate around effectively. This place-based reality resonates with Wayne Booth's discussion of the role of rhetoric as fundamental to reconciliation. The rhetoric of reconciliation reveals our principles and presuppositions about the world and its nature, our methods of discussion, and our expectations about the possibilities of reconciliation.[9] All of these elements are rooted in place, whether it be a specific classroom, the local school, the local region, whatever. To most effectively teach and learn in reconciling ways, we need to, as Gary Snyder writes, "choose to live in a place as a sort of visitor, or try to become an inhabitant" (Snyder 1995, 195).

Snyder, a poet and professor from California, writes that as we attend to local identity, we realize that the academy is not segregated from the community in which it lives, from its locale. For some academics, this is a difficult pill to swallow. Too many of us have shaped our identities as place-less, unaligned, objective. Some of us locate by memory, naming that school from which we graduated as if it were a place of identity. What this finally means is that our teaching is ungrounded except in abstract ideas. That un-orientation/nonlocated identity makes reconciliatory work impossible because there is no one *there* to work with or to do the work. The un-oriented has no stake, nothing to base a "how" upon. Reconciliatory practices cannot thrive in this setting. We must at least take seriously our classroom as a real place, a community, located and shaped by the identities, cultures, and content within it.

Within those walls are many other places, birth-lines, family heritages, racial identifications, classes, genders, communication and learning styles, and so forth. The place of our teaching and learning is inherently reconciliatory if one recognizes and takes seriously this location. How we teach will determine if the learning can tolerate the conflict, challenge, and mediated agreement inherent to this kind of place. Will we consciously adopt pedagogies that acknowledge and work with the reality of our classroom setting, at least? At most, we are teaching skills and knowledge that will help us and our students live daily in a civic modality attuned to reconciliation. We hope to shape communities within those walls that can connect with other communities beyond them in order to work for the common good (Erlich 1997, 62). But this perspective requires serious intention if it is to thrive. While learning theory and skills of analysis, we also are learning how to relate with others amid those ideas and practices. We must be able to bring information sensitive to audience, to various intentions, to different types of actions. We are looking to reach "beyond the minimal responsibilities of a citizen" (Erlich, 63).

Universities then, faculty, administrators, and staff, must begin to examine our place-based identities, assumptions, and preferred methods of living and learning as well as our cultural memories, experiences, and dynamics of power. We must acknowledge and respectfully share and examine our diverse backgrounds, life experiences, insights, and hopes in order to be known as ones inhabiting not only our campus but also our local communities. When we are clear about our place, our students will become clear and empowered as well. We develop rhetorics of place that locate us enough to have a moral and intellectual stake in how we can share a common ground in which all can fight, agree, thrive, move forward.

How can such a localized community of teachers and learners be created? What makes for such common ground while retaining our identity as academic institutions? How do we shape rhetorics of reconciliation specifically related to our particular arts of contestation, to quote Wayne Booth? What do we believe in and how did that come to be? What methods of discussion are most likely to yield reconciliation, knowing the histories and memories and dreams of our place? What is required of institutions that want to participate in this difficult and rewarding work? These are thick and difficult questions, certainly unanswerable in this short essay. However, I offer below some responses and hope the conversation will continue.

Shaping a Localized Community of Reconciliatory Teaching and Learning

I begin most of the classes I teach with introductions. I ask students to jot down a few notes about how their story, including their intellectual story, brought them to this class. What do they dread? What do they hope for and happily anticipate? Where do they see their learning taking them beyond this classroom? We then share our responses in small groups. Then I open it up for public comments about what folks learned, what they think about the responses, and what was surprising. I do this whether the class has eight students or forty-eight. I am still surprised to learn that at least a few have a refugee or immigrant background. Several are usually strongly identified with geographical regions and/or ethnic communities. Some have taken the class as an act of resistance—to family expectations, upbringing, and so on. I ask that everyone take notes on what we have heard and turn in by the next class a one-to-two-page reflective piece on "who we are as a class." I leave the format for this first assignment quite open because I have learned over the years that the students' choice of framing often tells me as much about them as the content. They are always stirred by each other's writings that are posted on our class's server, and this begins a pulse of energy that carries the class throughout the semester. That energy is potent for learning because students are taken out of themselves while sharing themselves. They name themselves while being drawn to others through the amazing diversity of reasons that people decided to take the class and what they hope to gain from and contribute to it.

This is a process of determining our initial landscape of inquiry and action as a class. Our boundaries are named, and usually during the second class I draw a comprehensive map on the board of who are, what we bring, and what we hope for, including where I see us going. We discuss this, but conclude nothing, instead noting points of convergence and divergence. Already we are recognizing how our stories, interests, and expectations will require collaboration, and perhaps even reconciliation, if we are to move forward toward shared learning goals.

If the class involves community-based teaching and learning, as does the Religion Internship course that I teach, I tell the story of how the class came to be community based. The narrative invariably catches the attention and imagination of the students. The internship class, for example, began through the intention of two professors from the Religion Department over twenty-one years ago. Who they were and what they stood for became one of the major legacies of our department, that of scholar-activist, first local and then global. This class, then, is part of that legacy—how will we fulfill that? One way we start is by overlaying our assets, ascertained from students' self-reporting, with the assets of various community organizations. Where are the matches of needs with assets, levers with difficult situations? This is reconciliatory work, merging stories and assets for shared purposes.[10]

The larger story, of course, is Emory University's story of engaged teaching and learning as scholarship. Often my students are surprised to discover that "their" Emory began in Oxford, Georgia, thirty miles south of Atlanta. The members of the Georgia Conference of the Methodist Episcopal Church founded a "Manual Training School." The vision for the school included the following:

> Manual labor shall be combined with literary instruction. . . . It is not designed to confine the labor of the pupils to agriculture alone, but to embrace the most common and profitable of the mechanic arts. . . . It is difficult to determine whether the poor, or the rich will be most benefited by this system of education; the indigent will be enabled to acquire an education, by them generally unattainable; the rich will form habits of industry, and self-dependence, more valuable than gold and silver; both may have vigorous and cultivated intellects in sound and healthy bodies, and learn to adapt the theories of science to the practical purposes of life. . . . (Ignatius Few in the *Southern Recorder*)

Suddenly, students are introduced to an unexpected history of and purpose in Emory's vision of education and the underlying religious values and character-forming practices to be embraced.

The roots of this place, Emory, resonate through the Georgia Methodists, with much of the democratizing goals of general American higher education. John Emory, the bishop for whom our school was named, wrote: "Education, properly, embraces the whole wide scope of the character, condition, and interests of man, physical, mental, moral, and religious for time and eternity."[11] From our very start at Emory, education was about holistic maturation in preparation for service now, with some eye toward eternity. Our classroom, though distinct and in an institution that had changed some over time, was also embedded in the particularities of this place and our founders' philosophies and methods.

Attempting to reconcile and integrate contested categories such as intellectual and pragmatic training, poor and rich, heart/mind and body, the Manual Labor School reported its successes every year at graduation. During the final graduation-type exercises, before it was totally folded into the newly emerging Emory College, the program listed twenty presentations by the students, including ten orations and several selections of vocal music. The topics of the orations ranged from "The American Colonies" to "Political Strife" to "Instability of Human Governments." The agricultural aspects of the school included plantings in cotton, corn, oats, wheat, and potatoes. Three hours a day were given to manual work, including farming or the mechanical trades. Faculty positions were Superintendent, Mathematics Teacher, Teacher of Languages, Farmer, Steward, and English Teacher.

Though the Manual Labor School might feel like prehistoric time to our class, its legacy affects us through continued values of the institution. I share other more recent quotes with the students indicating the purposes of this place. Bishop Warren Candler, who provided much of our twentieth-century leadership, is remembered as saying that education was for honor and usefulness. The usefulness to which he referred fit very well into the overall goal of being reconciling people, graduates engaged in community leadership based on their learning. The current mission statement of Emory continues the tradition:

> Emory University's mission is to create, preserve, teach, and apply knowledge in the service of humanity. . . . [This includes] a commitment to use knowledge to improve human well-being.[12]

This small sharing of history—building our class on the foundation of our school's history and values—helps students recognize that their learning is more than content. It is also purpose and meaning for the common good.

As with liberal arts colleges and research institutions all over America, there is a long tradition of education at Emory that emphasizes practical subjects and problem-solving skills. Engaging these skills enables students to also become "charged with theory and intellectual insight" (Erlich 1997, 63) as they experience the power of ideas in action. Reconciliatory teaching and learning have been part of the Emory University identity for over 150 years. When students can connect their hopes with these hopes, it is transformative for learning. The energy has coherence, a frame of meaning that is invaluable whether we embrace it, resist it, or reconstruct it.

Rhetoric and Methods of Reconciliatory Practices in Teaching and Learning

Creating community in a classroom by sharing stories and places and their inherent values highlights the conversational or dialogic nature of learning and teaching that is experientially based. A key aspect of an academic experience according to Thomas Erlich is "shared conversations of values and practices of communication, organization, compromise, participation, and change" (1997, 62). Rhetoric and communication, the bread and butter of teaching and learning, seem inherently involved with reconciliatory practices. Conversation is an art, and a tricky one at that, especially if you publicly recognize the diversity of those involved. To help our classroom conversations move toward shared goals, a few parameters for discussion are useful.

Usually early on in an experiential learning class, I give out a handout on skillful discussions. Taken from the insightful book *The Fifth Discipline: The Art and Practice of the Learning Organization* by Peter M. Senge, the handout states in short order steps for how to have an effective conversation that leads to a decision. The process reminds us as a class that any discussion if thick enough and serious enough involves ideas and negotiations. Learning to make decisions as a class is a paramount skill not only for our work, but also for work we do beyond our classroom walls. First, the handout reminds students to reflect initially on their own ideas, feelings, and goals before speaking. It reminds us also to listen carefully to the ideas of others and take them seriously. We are encouraged to ponder them before challenging or amending. If inner tensions arise, note if something the speaker said conflicts with your own ideas, feelings, and goals. If so, ask why. Listen to the answers that begin to emerge and work with them, internally and with others. Finally, move forward together toward sharpening the intended goal or decision you want, intellectually and pragmatically.

Attending to the inner conversation as well as the outer conversation makes for richer and deeper dialogue because there is increased awareness of and honesty about the push and pull of self, other, and place amid ideas and proposed actions. These dynamics are always present in reconciliatory work, and learning to recognize them sooner and more thoroughly can help any classroom think well. It also teaches us how to discern what must be addressed, what can wait, and/or what is "my problem" and why. These insights, which are intellectual as well as personal, help us decide together our common ground—what works and what makes sense. Having these guidelines in hand, we practice. I ask someone in the class each session to monitor our work and help us discover specific ways we can improve our negotiating practices. Working with the insights of skillful discussions, we test the steps and see if they open more possibilities for learning about and sharing ideas and theories. These assumptions, approaches, and feelings might not otherwise emerge nor be named in a less experience-oriented class. Nevertheless, these dynamics are at work, and they are crucial elements for reconciliatory practices. Recognizing them and working with them, though the work is hard, pays off. But it requires intention, structure, and practice.

In addition to skillful discussion practices, a class can increase its potential for reconciling work since it knows who has what skills in the class. These differences become more of our mapped assets, helping us more quickly turn to the right sources for analysis, theory building, hypothesis-creation, test-implementation, and so forth. We are learning how to communicate in the most effective ways the connections of ideas to plans, to actions. Who is patient? Who gets things done on time? As we continue to develop our skills, we become more adept at working together. Collaboration for change is easier, more accessible.

When students see themselves as agents, as owners and contributors in the process of shared learning and transformation, they increase their willingness to risk. Their imaginations are freed to explore other ways of knowing, different perspectives, other points of view. The energy of the class becomes identifiably communal, with a shared standpoint of joint respect built on intellectual and process skills. Eventually, a spontaneous process of shared work happens as students turn to particular members of the class, asking them to lead a discussion, or turn to others that they now know are more skilled in a particular form of analysis. The team has taken shape and the debates move forward more substantively and clearly. The challenge for the teacher, of course, is to ask students weaker in one area to apprentice themselves to another student who is more capable in those particular skills. Sometimes, of course, students resist this, preferring to stay in their better-known territory. But I emphasize with them that a reconciling approach in learning involves identifying one's strengths as well as one's weaknesses and then putting oneself in positions to practice with both while contributing to the common goals of the class.

Naturally as students feel more confidence and discover more agency, conversation not only increases but also becomes more contested and complex. Knowing more about their own and their classmates' assets, they also stretch and push each other toward more difficult territory. They argue. In fact, my classes often become quite heated. In one class, for example, the students were advanced in analysis and discussion, and they got into a major argument. The issue was race, and the question was who could claim that they were oppressed. A white male insisted that he experienced oppression and saw it in the white men he was serving in his community placement. Quickly, African Americans and women in the class revolted against his ideas, though they never attacked him personally. They used material we had been studying to challenge his remarks, and they could do this with complexity because they knew his story and his approaches to ideas and actions. They positioned his perception as outside the parameters of "real" oppression. The discussion became tense, and I found myself feeling increasingly anxious with the intensity, while also impressed at the students' ability to move through this contestation.

There was no final resolution that day, no notable reconciliation except that people kept their boundaries and their citizenship in the classroom community. They distinguished talking about themselves from the constituencies they served as well as from each other. I was pleased to hear them making connections within and beyond the classroom. Ideas were traveling, becoming bridges to their active work. Readings were quoted. Theories were applied. Yet, I remained unsettled after class at the strong words that were shared. I had noticed that some became quiet amid the strong voices. So I asked seven of the most vocal students to meet with me in my office a few days after this discussion. I told them of my concerns. They were silent for a while.

But then, the most involved African American man in the class looked directly at me and said, "Dr. Patterson, I really don't understand what's the big deal. You've been teaching us how to become an authentic, holistic learning community—as you call it. We've been working to bring all we have intellectually and humanely to our problem-solving work. So, we got into a fight? So, we got passionate?" The young white man who had begun the conversation quickly echoed him. They agreed that the work of reconciliatory learning and teaching so emphasized in our class was finally really engaged. We had done it. We had moved to the difficult, truly contested areas of our thinking and living. And the conversation had been a good one—moreover, a fair one. Another student agreed. Then another and another. Thanks to them, I began to reconcile myself to the reality that we had in fact created a space in which struggle and tense dialogue were safe and very real—meaning, it touched living issues that mattered deeply to all involved, both personally and in their work beyond the classroom. We had kept our boundaries and our skills, and had begun to think together in order to act. Finally, we were in a class living ideas, not just thinking them.

Contested ideas are, of course, the heart of teaching and learning in any flourishing context. But I find that this engaged level of dialogue is often missing from classrooms. Ideas do not matter enough, perhaps, because they are not quite connected enough with the real issues of our lives. But with attention to connecting ideas and experiences, students quickly learn to press each other whether negotiating common ground or not. Yet amid the push and pull, there are reconciling moments of simply being heard, of being taken seriously enough to be challenged or even denied, of having your idea worked with and/or perhaps reconstructed in order to gel with others on the table. The proof of these reconciliatory practices is in the relative ease with which I watch students accept the rejection of their ideas by their peers. They report that in this environment it is easier to listen, to let go, or to negotiate. They know the process of discussion guarantees that they will be taken seriously even if finally rejected. Hopefully as we teachers become more comfortable with these pedagogical approaches, we too will relax and enjoy the passion of our students as we move forward in our reconciliatory work.

What I have learned over the years at Emory is that ideas about reconciliatory teaching and learning have concrete consequences. Ideas become living experiences in the classroom that are connected to real people and their real concerns in and beyond the walls we share. Classrooms can become localized generators of reconciliatory teaching and learning on many levels and in many ways. It may be that reconciliatory work comes through arguments over the interpretation of a text, or the incompatibility of a reading in relation to the active engagement of it beyond the classroom. Reconciliatory practices may arise as different kinds of experiences bring alternative views of what the text assumes in order to come to its conclusions. The point of contestation in a reconciliatory environment is to offer students the opportunity to identify a problem, to know how to work independently and interdependently on it, and to determine ways of resolving it collaboratively and respectfully for all involved.

The shift is discipline-based learning to interdisciplinary problem-solving in the service of reconciliation as widely defined and as locally lived as possible. Through arguments and debate, students practice useful methods of discussion and structured reflection about the processes appropriate for responding in holistic and transformative ways to a problem.[13] Whether the arguments are rooted in theoretical discussion, community-based service, or participatory action research for community-driven change, the work of the classroom is to provide practices to the students that serve reconciliatory responses.

The Rewards and Tensions of Reconciliatory Practices of Teaching and Learning

Reconciliatory practices of teaching and learning are, of course, present in any classroom whether attended to or not. But they can be engaged fruitfully if acknowledged and structured intentionally for specific learning goals. They are more easily worked with in experientially based classes. The joys of watching students engage a topic not only intellectually but also pragmatically makes one remember why one accepted this vocation in the first place. It is no wonder that active teaching and learning strategies are being increasingly used across the country. But we need more models, and more analysis and critiques of the ones we are currently using—a reconciliatory practice in itself.

The complex realities of our world place new demands on how and why we teach and learn. How can we effectively build on the legacy of reconciliatory education in America? Surely we need to create students familiar with the intellectual and pragmatic practices of transforming violence and stagnation into positive change for the common good—however that contested term is mediated. Because the meanings and enactments of reconciliation continually change, our pedagogical models need an openness that can create flexible teachers and learners able to hear, speak, and act across boundaries of culture, context, story, category, and academic discipline. We must live with the ongoing tensions, acknowledging them in our classrooms, rather than avoiding them. We need strategies for addressing difficulties in creating partnerships, distorted understandings, confused and deadly fears, dramatic sources of hopefulness in theory and action, genuine communication and action. We must examine and practice these as part of our learning agenda. This is the challenge before us.

To engage in this project from a reconciliatory view, we gain insight from John Dewey's pragmatism emphasizing teaching students to focus on data collection, followed by integrative analysis and critical thinking that become engaged citizenship (Erlich 1997, 62). It will also require that teachers from many different disciplines join hands to provide students with all the resources and expertise that they need. There needs to be civil respect and communication among different departments of the school, serious cooperation across disciplines that is not seen as added on to an existing teaching and research load, but accepted as appropriately part of it. Tensions around funding and territory will need to be debated publicly, a reconciliatory practice of its own and one with which the academy is generally unfamiliar and unpracticed.

Serious recognition of the scholarship of teaching along the lines of creating the next generation of scholar citizens prepared for reconciliatory work is not a fantasy. There are resources within and beyond the academy. Taking community knowledge seriously will be an important step. There needs to be a new level of shared power and decision making in joint ventures with local groups. Some universities, such as the University of Pennsylvania, have built on existing community–university relationships in order to solve problems that are of mutual concern. Neighborhood residents and school personnel from West Philadelphia joined in partnership with Penn to create the West Philadelphia Improvement Corps (WEPIC). Together they committed to transform the neighborhood that was visibly deteriorating in infrastructure, economy, and education with additional consequences for the university. Together they planned to bring requested strategic assistance from Penn students, faculty, and staff to help transform the traditional West Philadelphia public school system into a "revolutionary" new system of university-assisted, community-developing, community-centered, community resource-mobilizing, community problem-solving, schools (Harkavay and Puckett 1991; Harkavay and Benson 2002). The mutually agreed-upon decision was to begin by focusing on having an achievable, visible, and dramatic success in one school. The result has been a variety of ongoing activities focusing on the interactive relationships among diet, nutrition, growth, and health as contributing to a flourishing life for children in the school. The program has been a great success, and Penn believes that the moral and intellectual development of the undergraduates involved has been of equal success (Harkavay and Benson 2002, 17).

Such initiatives will also necessitate increased communication among faculty, students, and trustees as partners working together toward common goals with a willingness to seriously negotiate long-held assumptions and resources. Such commitments must be long-term and continually discussed. They are best stabilized when related to the founding missions of an institution and supported by the top officers of the school. The legacy of American higher education must be more fully engaged again with resources given from an agreed-upon commitment by all involved. The assumption that becomes reality is that the university is willing to stake its intellectual work in the daily push and pull of negotiating a better world for us all. Surely 9/11 demonstrated again the fact that we who teach and learn must discover strategies of inquiry and practices of vision that can create and achieve reconciliation in our own day.

Notes

1. An article that provided our framework for thinking about method and methodology is by Jon R. Stone in an edited volume, *The Craft of Religious Studies*, pages 1–17.

2. For more reading in this area, see David Kolb's *Experiential Learning: Experience as the Source of Learning and Development*, and Howard Gardner's *Frames of Mind*.

3. A complete discussion of the content, skill, attitudinal, and behavioral outcomes of service learning as holistic learning can be found in Janet Eyler and Dwight Giles, *Where Is the Learning in Service Learning*. The book is a comprehensive study of students from many different schools and programs across the United States that use experiential/service learning approaches.

4. The section of the book that is particularly pertinent to these processes is found on pages 171–191.

5. Dr. Patricia Killen of Pacific Lutheran University taught this sequencing pattern at a two-day workshop on teaching and learning at Emory.

6. Janet Eyler of Vanderbilt University developed this multidimensional outcome of experiential learning.

7. Ira Harkavay gave these quotations during his presentation at the Sam Nunn Policy Forum co-sponsored by the Ethics Center of Emory University during 1999.

The title of the forum was "Citizenship for a New Millennium" and the focus was on leadership and values. For additional information, see other materials co-written by Harkavay in the bibliography.

8. The Kellogg Foundation's new initiative for higher education is called "The Engaged University."

9. See Wayne Booth, *The Vocation of a Teacher: Rhetorical Occasions.*

10. For more complete understanding of community change through asset identification and resourcing, see John Kretzmann and John McKnight, *Building Communities from the Inside Out.*

11. Robert Emory, *Life of the Rev. John Emory* (D.D. New York: George Lane, 1841) p. 285. My deep appreciation goes to Ginger Cain, Emory University archivist, for her insights into Emory's founding.

12. For the complete mission statement of Emory University, see www.emory.edu/PRESIDENT/mission.html.

13. Joseph Cadray, a professor of the Education Department at Emory, brought to my attention an excellent article on reflective processes and teaching and learning by Edward P. St. John and Larry D. Burlew (see bibliography).

Bibliography

Arendt, Hannah. 1958. *The Human Condition.* Chicago: University of Chicago Press.

Booth, Wayne C. 1988. *The Vocation of a Teacher: Rhetorical Occasions.* Chicago: University of Chicago Press.

Boyer, Ernest L. 1990. *Scholarship Reconsidered: Priorities of the Professoriate.* Princeton, NJ: Carnegie Foundation for the Advancement of Teaching.

Checkoway, Barry. 1997. "Reinventing the Research University for Public Service." *Journal of Planning Literature* 11, 3: 307–318.

Erlich, Thomas. 1997. "Civic Learning: Democracy and Education Revisited." *Educational Record* (Summer–Fall): 57–65.

Eyler, Janet. 1995. "Comparing the Impact of Two Internship Experiences on Student Learning." *Journal of Cooperative Education* 29, 3: 41–52.

Eyler, Janet, and Dwight E. Giles. 1999. *Where Is the Learning in Service Learning?* San Francisco: Jossey-Bass.

Gardner, Howard. 1983. *Frames of Mind: The Theory of Multiple Intelligences.* New York: BasicBooks of HarperCollins.

Harkavay, Ira, and Lee Benson. 2002. "The Role of Community–Higher Education School Partnerships in Educational and Social Development and Democratization." In *Universities and Community Schools* 7, 1–2 (Fall–Winter): 6–28 (Philadelphia: University of Pennsylvania).

Harkavay, Ira, and John L. Puckett. 1991. "The Role of Mediating Structures in University Community Revitalization: The University of Pennsylvania and West Philadelphia as a Case Study." *Journal of Research and Development in Education* 25, 1: 10–25.

Kegan, Robert. 1994. *In Over Our Heads: The Mental Demands of Modern Life.* Cambridge, MA: Harvard University Press.

Kolb, David L. 1984. *Experiential Learning: Experience as the Source of Learning and Development.* Englewood Cliffs, NJ: Prentice Hall.

Kretzmann, John P., and John L. McKnight. 1993. *Building Communities from the Inside Out: A Path Toward Finding and Mobilizing a Community's Assets*. Chicago: ACTA Publications.

St. John, Edward P., and Larry D. Burlew. 1993. "A Developmental Perspective on Reflective Practice: An Application of Jung's Theory of Individuation." *Louisiana Journal of Counseling* 4, 1: 9–24.

Senge, Peter M. 1990. *The Fifth Discipline: The Art and Practice of the Learning Organization*. New York: Doubleday.

Snyder, Gary. 1995. *A Place in Space: Ethics, Aesthetics, and Watersheds*. Washington, DC: Counterpoint Press.

Stone, Jon R., ed. 1998. *The Craft of Religious Studies*. New York: St. Martin's.

September 11 and the Search for Justice and Accountability

Abdullahi Ahmed An-Na'im

People scarred by violence and injustice tend to turn to vigilante justice or other nonlegal means to address an intolerable situation. The current Islamic jihad, or holy war, declared by Osama bin Laden and al-Qaeda, is one example of an aggressive attempt at "self-help" that spurns legal remedies. Because this view of jihad and vigilante justice is morally repugnant and pragmatically untenable, we must invest in structures to support viable and sustainable reconciliation. I am calling in particular for the development of the necessary normative and institutional resources for continuing reconciliation.

Terrorism's Past and Future

What concerns me most as a Muslim advocate of peace and reconciliation is the "Islamic dimension" of the terrorists' attacks of September 11, 2001, although I do not at all suggest that this is the only, or even primary, feature of those tragic events. The atrocities of September 11 are commonly attributed to a terrorist network known as al-Qaeda, under the leadership of Osama bin Laden (who claimed responsibility for similar attacks on American embassies in Nairobi, Kenya, and Dar es Salaam, Tanzania, in August 1998). The reality of an international terrorist network that claims an Islamic rationale for its activities calls into question the nature and implications of the doctrine of jihad under Shari'a (the normative law of Islam).

The Arabic term *jihad* simply means self-exertion or special effort, and is used in the Qur'an to refer to a variety of senses, including combating one's illegitimate desires, and to activities undertaken in peaceful propagation of the faith.[1] But the term is also used in the Qur'an and in Islamic jurisprudence in general to signify religiously sanctioned use of force either in self-defense or to propagate or "defend" the faith. This latter sense of jihad clearly conflicts with the principles of reconciliation because it sanctions direct and unregulated violent action in pursuit of political objectives at the risk of harm to innocent bystanders.

The relationship between Shari'a and direct violent action in pursuit of what someone deems to be legitimate objectives has been a highly contested subject among Muslims since the first civil war (al-Fitnah al-Kubra) following the rebellion against Uthman, the third Caliph, and his murder in 656 C.E., only twenty-four years after the death of the Prophet Mohammed.[2] On one hand, the personal obligation of every Muslim to uphold justice and combat injustice, regardless of what the wider community or state is willing or able to do, can have obvious social and political merit. On the other hand, there would be total chaos if each Muslim were simply to act on his or her own initiative in redressing what he or she deems to be injustice, without resort to lawful authorities charged with maintaining public peace and order. This profound ambivalence to political violence cannot be resolved on purely theological grounds, as Islamic scriptural sources can be cited in support of each side of the controversy. As I have argued elsewhere, however, these competing textual sources can only be understood and reconciled with reference to a contextual framework for their meaning and practical application at different times in history.[3]

The ambivalence of Shari'a about the use of force in national politics and international relations is understandable in the harsh and violent context of its origins and early development in the seventh to ninth centuries, where use of force was the unquestioned norm. In fact, Shari'a represented an improvement in that context by limiting the legitimate use of force to self-defense and propagation of Islam, though the latter rationale was in fact used to achieve territorial expansion of Islamic states throughout history. Shari'a also regulated the conduct of hostilities, including the requirement of what might be called a formal declaration of war in modern usage and the strict prohibition of killing children, old men, women, and noncombatants.[4] In this light, it can fairly be concluded that the attacks of 9/11 violated Shari'a principles on the legitimate use of force in international relations. But it is also true to say that there is an underlying ambivalence in those principles that may lead some Muslims to believe themselves justified in the use of such arbitrary and unregulated violence in pursuit of political objectives or under an expansive notion of self-defense. If and when those Muslims believe that there is no redress to grave injustice under the rule of law—what I call here normative and institutional resources for reconciliation—they may invoke a religious justification for direct violent action against what they regard as corrupt governments at home or perceived enemies abroad.[5]

Turning to the American side, I find that one of the clear lessons of the atrocities of 9/11 is a fundamental sense of shared vulnerability, in that all human beings everywhere are vulnerable to arbitrary violence. This point was tragically illustrated by the crude manner in which nineteen determined terrorists were able to inflict the horrendous carnage and destruction of 9/11 in the heartland of the most powerful country in the world. The trauma of the attacks was compounded by the scale and speed by which the terrorists managed to shatter the illusion of security and predictability of daily life where that was most certainly taken for granted. It is imperative to appreciate the wide variety of ways in which all human beings everywhere experience this shared vulnerability. For some, it is the threat of terrorism and other forms of political violence; for others it is political oppression, religious or ethnic persecution, or poverty and disease. The challenge is to see the connections between all these forms of vulnerability so that we can realize that addressing one form can help alleviate another. In relation to 9/11 in particular, we need to realize that addressing the grievances of the terrorists over the Israeli/Palestinian conflict or perceptions of American complicity in the political and economic frustration in some countries can reduce the risk of terrorist attacks. To say this is not to condone terrorism in the least, but only to acknowledge the rationality of the terrorists, though we disagree with their logic, conclusion, and methods.

The strength of the fallacy that one nation could be exempt from this universally shared vulnerability of human beings is reflected in the profound loss of personal security many people feel in the post–September 11 environment in United States. Paradoxically, in the aftermath of that tragedy, many citizens of the United States seemed to cling to the illusion of invulnerability by granting their government extraordinary powers to do whatever it deems necessary against this new, amorphous, and invisible danger. In addition to failing to critically evaluate the relationship between such excessive powers and the achievement of the desired objective, this attitude raises the serious risk of severe and irreversible loss of the same liberties and values it seeks to safeguard. On one hand, the limitations of human and material resources and time constraints, as well as inevitable complacency and bureaucratic inertia, would tend to limit the practical efficacy of such measures in combating terrorism. On the other hand, in monitoring and tracking the movements and activities of potential terrorists within the United States, the government will necessarily harass and intrude on the privacy of countless innocent citizens and lawful residents.[6]

Such a simplistic approach to the threat of terrorism, and abdication of responsibility by citizens of the most powerful nation in the world, fails to appreciate that events like 9/11 always have a past and a future. Again, without in the least condoning those atrocious attacks, an appropriate response to them would attempt to understand the motivation of the terrorists, however unjustified one may believe it to be, as well as take into consideration the likely consequences of the actions of the government of the United States in retaliation. As former President Jimmy Carter has said:

> We have ignored or condoned abuses in nations that support our anti-terrorism effort, while detaining American citizens as "enemy combatants," incarcerating them secretly and indefinitely without their being charged with any crime or having the right to legal counsel. This policy has been condemned by the federal courts, but the Justice Department seems adamant, and the issue is still in doubt. Several hundred captured Taliban soldiers remain imprisoned at Guantanamo Bay under the same circumstances, with the defense secretary declaring that they would not be released even if they were someday tried and found to be innocent. These actions are similar to those of abusive regimes that historically have been condemned by American presidents.[7]

An understanding of the history and consideration for the future would clearly indicate the futility of lawless unilateral retaliation at the presumed source of harm, without addressing the underlying causes that apparently prompted the perpetrators to commit their heinous crimes and may persuade others to condone or facilitate similar violence. The fact that a hard-core group of religious, ideological extremists like those who perpetrated the terrorist attacks will probably harbor aggressive designs without justification does not mean that their grievances should never be taken seriously, since some of them may indeed be shared by more reasonable people who can be influenced by appropriate action. Since hard-core elements cannot act out their aggression without the support, or at least acquiescence, of a larger number of people who are open to reason and humanitarian concern, the sensibilities and grievances of those wider constituencies must be seriously addressed. Recalling the coincidence of moral and pragmatic considerations noted earlier, addressing the grievances of that wider constituency is both morally required and pragmatically necessary in order to deny terrorists that source of moral and material support.

Twin Pillars of Reconciliation: Justice and Accountability

Reconciliation is a constant process whose outcome is contingent upon various factors but always requires building consensus across cultural and ideological boundaries. The twin pillars of a successful and sustainable process of reconciliation, in my view, are justice and accountability. Justice addresses the underlying causes of that desperate and lawless behavior, and accountability addresses the violation of the rule of law in international and national affairs. Both elements, however, require consensus on the normative and institutional resources that undergird the rationale of the process of reconciliation.

My analysis rests on three propositions about the process of reconciliation. First, it is neither possible nor desirable to permanently eliminate difference or conflict in human relationships at all levels, from the personal to the national and international. Instead of assuming that the core of the conflict is in its immediate expression, it should be seen as a natural phenomenon, which "transforms events, the relationships with which conflict occurs, and indeed its very creators."[8] Conflict facilitates social, personal, and communal transformations and growth, which, in turn, modify the immediate expression of conflict, as well as the people, context, and relationships involved. Thus, "neither social forces [like entrepreneurs, workers, students, women, and peasants] nor social movements [whether ethnic, religious, national liberation, etc.] can be presumed to have an internal consistency and coherence, or be the agent of realizing a trans-historical agenda."[9] It is therefore important to build on possibilities of agreement across presumed dividing lines, instead of assuming total homogeneity on either side of a conflict.

Second, all human beings, as individuals or in groups, live by the moral and pragmatic choices they make, whether made actively and consciously or passively and subconsciously. Failing to make a choice for change is a choice by default that tends to support the status quo, whatever it may be. Moreover, while individual choices are often made in response or reaction to choices made by others, each actor at every stage has the possibility and ability to make a different response. For example, the fact that X hit Y does not necessarily compel or require Y to hit back in retaliation, as Y may well decide that self-restraint is in his own best interest in view of his personal assessment of the situation and its consequences.

Third, it is futile to expect people to make the moral and pragmatic choices in favor of reconciliation without securing their vital interests or addressing their own concerns and apprehensions. In the simplified example above, Y is less likely to hit back in retaliation if there are alterative means for holding X accountable for the initial attack, or for protecting Y against further aggression by X or any other person. Consequently, the viability and sustainability of reconciliation in continuing, multifaceted conflicts needs to draw upon normative and institutional resources for justice and accountability. The existence of fair and credible norms and mechanisms of accountability reduces the risk of self-help and vigilante justice. Conversely, resorting to self-help in retaliation against aggression tends to undermine the possibility of establishing a normative and institutional basis for fair and credible accountability. In other words, direct retaliation tends to perpetuate a vicious cycle of attack and counterattack, which diminishes the prospects of viable and sustainable reconciliation among the parties to conflict. But since a different choice is always available to all sides in a conflict, each side can seek to break that cycle anytime, which is more likely to happen when there are prospects of justice and accountability.

To briefly elaborate on these three propositions, I would first emphasize that the maxim noted in the Introduction of this volume—"there can be no peace without justice"—immediately raises at least two questions about the meaning and practical implementation of justice and accountability. Since people tend to have different conceptions of justice in any given context, the first question is how to promote consensus on understandings of justice. Moreover, since such consensus is unlikely to be achieved without a framework for dialogue among competing perspectives, and cannot be sustained over time without credible accountability for violating its precepts, the second question is how to regulate these necessary processes. As I see it, reconciliation requires an institutional framework for dialogue to develop normative agreement among the parties about a just mediation of their differences, as well as mechanisms for the constant adjudication of disputes. This framework must also ensure accountability for violations of the agreed norms for regulating their relationship.

One point to emphasize about this vision is that the institutional framework for consensus-building, as well as accountability for its violation, must be founded on the same principles of justice agreed upon among the parties to a given conflict. The relationship between these ends and means should be seen as a continuum, from the structural forms and processes of institutions to the substantive outcomes of those forms and processes. This organic and dialectic relationship between procedural and substantive justice means that neither can be achieved without the other.

Furthermore, the need for normative and institutional resources for justice and accountability should be both prospective and reactive—reaching toward the future as well as the past. Assurances against future violations of the agreed norms of justice are probably more important to the continuing process of reconciliation than the satisfaction a victim may draw from exacting vengeance or punishment for past wrongs. This is not to say that one should never pursue accountability for past wrongs, as that may indeed be necessary and conducive to reconciliation in some cases. Rather, my point is that making reliable arrangements for future accountability is critical in all cases, regardless of whether or not accountability for past wrongs is sought or achieved. Moreover, this accountability may take the form of a wide variety of responses: truth-telling, acknowledgement of and apology for wrongdoing, appropriate restitution and reparation measures, and/ or punishment of the offender.

Finally, the analysis and conclusions of this essay are not intended to disregard or underestimate the difficulties and complexities of mediation and reconciliation of conflict. As the tragic events in the former Yugoslavia and Rwanda during the 1990s illustrate, there is often an atmosphere of distrust and misunderstanding that is heightened by memories of historical or recent atrocities. With charges and counter-charges about past events, there seems to be no constructive space in the history of the conflict for effective negotiations to occur. Yet, favorable conditions must somehow be established for the process to occur. Difficulties to be dealt with include: opposition or backlash from some factions on both sides, persistence of incompatible goals and lack of political progress, re-politicization of peace-building initiatives, and lack of human and material resources for implementing various strategies and programs. Moreover, there is always the question of how to make the whole process of reconciliation sustainable, by moving it from creating a conducive environment to maintaining human relationships, and generally building on the momentum of the conflict transformation. Giving due regard to such difficulties and complexities requires the recognition of reconciliation as a "process" rather than an event. For the same reason, we should realize that institutional and normative arrangements are only resources that may or may not result in the actual achievement of sustainable reconciliation on the ground.

International Law and Human Rights as Resources for Justice

These reflections on 9/11 and its aftermath lead me to the same conclusion about the imperative need for consensus on normative and institutional resources for reconciliation. On the Muslim side, there is need for an authoritative and principled rejection of any religious justification for unilateral preemptive or retaliatory violence, which will only legitimize a similar response by the other side. This transformation will require courageous and visionary leadership to advance the theological, social, and political case for change, in addition to confidence in the possibilities of peaceful and effective redress for the grievances of those Muslims who may be tempted to engage in terrorist attacks or to condone and support such conduct. On the American side, an appropriate response to the threat of international terrorism must be firmly grounded in a clear and profound appreciation of the multifaceted, universally shared vulnerability of all human beings. That appreciation would clearly exclude resort to unilateral preemptive or retaliatory violence, which will only legitimize the arbitrary lawlessness of the terrorist. In view of the understandable outrage and strong demands for retaliation for the 9/11 attacks, a reconciliatory approach would require courageous and visionary leadership at home, and the realistic prospect of redress and safeguards against further attacks abroad.

In other words, both sides need to engage in an internal process of transformation of their positions. This process cannot be initiated and sustained in the absence of normative and institutional resources for reconciliation of conflict. Proponents of reconciliation on both sides of this conflict need to rely on the plausibility of that process in the concrete realities of international relations. Muslim advocates of peaceful coexistence and reconciliation need to rely on the plausible reality and efficacy of the process of reconciliation according to agreed normative and institutional arrangements in their opposition to the negative and regressive notion of jihad that is manipulated by the terrorists to legitimize their unilateral and arbitrary direct violence. Similarly, American advocates of self-restraint and peaceful reconciliation cannot succeed politically without realistic prospects of securing accountability for 9/11 and credible safeguards against future threats to the security of their population and the sovereignty of their country.

Fortunately, we do have the necessary normative and institutional resources, namely, the principles and mechanisms of international law and human rights. I will now briefly review the principles and institutions that are relevant to each side of this conflict, as they may work in a possible process of reconciliation. However, the following review is not intended to be exhaustive or authoritative, but merely illustrative of the sort of normative and institutional resources that are available for reconciliation in this case. In particular, this review is subject to two caveats:

1. I am concerned here with establishing a general framework for the process of reconciliation, rather than the precise terms of legal responsibility of individual persons or states. Accordingly, I would readily concede that the relevance or application of some of the principles I am citing below can be disputed as a technical matter under international law. My objective is to make the case for getting the parties to a stage where such technical issues can be properly debated or adjudicated, rather than claiming to settle those issues in this limited space. For example, the definition of "crimes against humanity" I am relying on draws on sources that may not apply to the 9/11 situation, in a strict legal sense, but can be taken to be evidence of customary international law that would be applicable. Thus, the fact that the Rome Statute of the International Criminal Court does not apply to the terrorists in this case does not preclude citing that statute as indicating a definition of this crime under customary international law that is binding on all states, regardless of the coming into force of a particular treaty or that it has not been ratified by the states concerned.

2. The fact that the principles and institutions indicated below sound idealistic, perhaps even far-fetched, is part of my thesis in this essay. That is, a commitment to the process of reconciliation in international conflicts like 9/11 should include full acceptance of these principles and institutions as a matter of course. At the same time, however, I would not expect the concerned parties to immediately act in full accordance with these principles or submit to the jurisdiction of relevant institutions. As with the first caveat, the object here is to get the parties to the point where they would debate these issues in a peaceful and orderly manner, instead engaging in unilateral and arbitrary violence.

Based on publicly available news reports and media analysis,[10] I suggest that the attacks of 9/11 were committed by individuals and do not constitute an act of war by any state. As such, those attacks constitute crimes against humanity under international law,[11] in addition to any crimes committed under the federal and state jurisdictions of the United States. However, any state that harbors individuals responsible for committing, instigating, or aiding and abetting the commission of those crimes is responsible for either prosecuting those persons or handing them over for trial by a state that has jurisdiction.[12] Moreover, any persons arrested or detained on suspicion of being implicated on those crimes must receive the full protection and benefits of due process of law and requirements of a fair trial.[13]

In pursuing its legitimate right to justice and accountability for those crimes against humanity, the United States was and is bound by relevant principles of customary international law and the provisions of the Charter of the United Nations. These would include, for example, the obligation to refrain from the use of force against the territorial integrity or political independence of any state, and to settle international disputes by peaceful means in such a manner that international peace and security and justice are not endangered.[14] Moreover, the United States was and is bound by customary international law principles and specific treaties that regulate its treatment of any persons detained in the course of military operations or arrested on suspicion of commission of crimes. These would include provisions for the treatment of prisoners of war, as well as due process and fair trial requirements for criminal suspects.[15]

Drawing on this small sample of relevant principles of international law and human rights, a "best-case scenario" might have been for Islamic countries to strongly support the United States in pursuing a law enforcement model in seeking to identify and prosecute those individual persons who are responsible for the terrorist attacks of 9/11.[16] Given the necessary political will, I believe that enough normative and institutional resources exist to hold criminals accountable under international law, as illustrated by authoritative precedents, such as the successful prosecution in the Netherlands of Libyan nationals accused of the destruction of a Pan Am flight over Lockerbie, Scotland, in 1988.

If that option seemed too unrealistic in view of the political situation in the United States at the time, or if it was tried and failed, it would have been better to secure the authorization of the Security Council of the United Nations for U.S. military operations in Afghanistan (regardless of the possibility of the technical legality of that intervention, such as the pretext of being "invited" by the Northern Alliance as the nominal government of country). Unfortunately, the Security Council apparently seemed to abdicate its responsibility at the time by neither sanctioning nor condemning the military campaign of the United States in Afghanistan.[17] Space does not permit further examination of what has actually happened since 9/11. But as I emphasized earlier, it is never too late to try to initiate a reconciliation process. With this possibility in mind, I will now briefly summarize the current situation and its implications for reconciliation among the parties to this conflict.

Breaking the Cycle of Violence

To imagine the possibility of reconciliation and its requirements, one has to start at some point in the cycle of violence and counterviolence to consider what it would take to bring the parties to appreciating the need for reconciliation and having confidence in its viability and sustainability. To recall the main relevant elements of the aftermath of the 9/11 terrorist attacks, the United States launched a massive military campaign in Afghanistan on October 7, 2001, with the declared objective of destroying al-Qaeda, a network of international terrorists lead by Osama bin Laden, and overthrowing the Taliban government for having harbored and supported that network in its repeated attacks against the United States and its citizens. As noted earlier, although the United States was supported in that campaign by a number of allies, including several predominantly Muslim countries in Southern and Central Asia, that military action was neither sanctioned nor opposed by the Security Council of the United Nations.

The Taliban regime was overthrown by a combination of American and Northern Alliance forces within weeks of the initiation of that campaign, and a new government was instituted in Afghanistan by the end of 2001. However, with escape of the leadership and an unknown number of the members of al-Qaeda, including bin Laden himself and his main lieutenants, according to media reports, the U.S. military campaign in Afghanistan does not appear to have been as effective as hoped in achieving its primary goal of destroying the terrorist network.

Several months into that process, however, the United States suddenly shifted its main focus from the campaign against al-Qaeda and its affiliates to plans for a military invasion of Iraq, with the purported rationale shifting between the need to dismantle the country's weapons of mass destruction and removing the regime of Saddam Hussein in order to bring democracy to the Iraqi people. Whatever one may think of the reasons or basis of that action, Iraq was in fact invaded and occupied by the United States and the United Kingdom by April 2003. This happened not only without the sanction of the Security Council of the United Nations, but with the globally publicized knowledge that authorization for the invasion of Iraq was being authoritatively rejected by the Security Council. The strong majority of the members of the Council, including China, France, and Russia, who have the power to veto a resolution, insisted on granting weapons inspectors more time to search for weapons of mass destruction in Iraq.

Several aspects of the invasion and occupation of Iraq made it inevitable that it would be perceived as an effort to colonize the country. The United Kingdom, the primary partner of the United States in this invasion and occupation, was in fact the last European colonial power in Iraq, following the collapse of the Ottoman Empire after the end of World War I. The recent occupation is in effect colonization because it is the usurpation of the sovereignty of the country through military conquest, hence the rush, as this essay goes to press, by the United States to restore the "sovereignty" of Iraq by the end of June 2004. Like earlier episodes of colonialism in Africa and Asia, this occupation was rationalized in the name of establishing democracy, the current version of the "white man's burden" of nineteenth century colonialism. The perception of motives of colonial exploitation are further strengthened by the complete failure of the United States and the United Kingdom to either find weapons of mass destruction in Iraq or establish evidence of links between the regime of Saddam Hussein and al-Qaeda, the purported justifications for the invasion in the first place.

On the positive side, however, this colonial misadventure has clearly failed not only because of growing resistance by Iraqis, but also because of a continued and categorical rejection by international public opinion, including the opinion of some citizens of the United States and the United Kingdom. The occupying powers are clearly unable to maintain basic law and order or to provide essential services in many parts of the country, let alone promote democratic government in the face of continuing civil protests and mounting political complexity. In the end, the United States and Britain have had to resort to the United Nations to negotiate the "restoration" of Iraqi sovereignty, thereby reaffirming the supremacy of the same international legal body they undermined in their unilateral and unjustified invasion. I am therefore heartened and encouraged by the recent developments that support the thesis and analysis I have argued here.

As these developments continue to unfold, the original "war on international terrorism" in response to 9/11 is apparently receding into the background, except for various legal, diplomatic, and sometimes military actions being taken against suspected terrorists who are assumed to be affiliated with al-Qaeda. At the same time, news reports indicate that members of the network have regrouped in various countries in South and Southeast Asia and begun issuing new threats of violent attacks against American targets. Recent violent attacks on citizens of the United States and its Western allies, from Bali, Indonesia, to Riyadh, Saudi Arabia, are widely assumed to be perpetrated by al-Qaeda or its affiliates in various parts of the world.

The object of the preceding brief summary of the state of the conflict between the United States and the al-Qaeda network at the time of writing is not to settle the facts beyond dispute or allocate responsibility. Rather, my purpose is to use this outline to illustrate how a possible application of the principles of reconciliation discussed above might apply to this conflict. The underlying thesis of those principles, as emphasized at the beginning of this short essay, is that reconciliation should be seen as a continuous process that draws on normative and institutional resources for justice and accountability. This thesis is premised on the following propositions:

- Conflict is a permanent feature of all human relationships.
- All human beings live by the moral and pragmatic choices they make or fail to make, but a different choice is always possible.

- To assist people in opting for reconciliation, their vital security and concerns must be addressed through fair and credible norms and mechanisms of accountability.

Applying this thesis and its premise to 9/11 and its aftermath, the United States is clearly entitled to accountability for the terrorist attacks, in addition to effective measures to ensure respect for its sovereignty, protection of the security of its territory, and safety of its citizens. As suggested earlier, however, those objectives could have been pursued through a law enforcement approach, instead of the massive military attacks against Afghanistan and Iraq, which resulted in the deaths of several thousand civilians and the radicalization of the mainstream Muslim public opinion. Such negative consequences not only entrench the position of the Islamic terrorists, but also give them the sympathy and support of many who would have otherwise condemned terrorism as inhumane and counterproductive.

Even if the law enforcement approach was politically impossible or practically ineffective in this case, military action under the auspices of the UN Security Council would have been more consistent with a process of reconciliation. But since that course of action was not taken either, as noted earlier, the question now is, how can reconciliation work? Here is how I believe it possible to move the process forward:

It is clear that the leadership and membership of the al-Qaeda network will not submit to accountability under international law, or under the domestic law of any country that may have jurisdiction over them. But it is equally clear that al-Qaeda and other terrorist organizations cannot exist, let alone effectively operate, without the substantial material and moral support of a much larger number of sympathetic Muslims. Reconciliation efforts should therefore address that much wider network of support, rather than the hard-core terrorists who will never listen to reason or be moved by humanitarian concerns. But that wider Muslim public may now be further alienated by the conduct of the United States in Afghanistan and Iraq, in addition to traditional concerns about the legitimate rights of the Palestinians and U.S. support of oppressive regimes in the region.

In my view, the most effective way to move the majority of Muslims toward reconciliation is for the United States to declare its complete commitment to observe international law and respect human rights in its pursuit of accountability for 9/11 and security against future terrorist attacks. Without such a categorical affirmation of the rule of law in international relations, reasonable and fair-minded Muslims would have no conceptual or political reasons for renouncing the traditional doctrine of jihad that is used by terrorists to gain public support for their actions. But the United States may also be unwilling to make this commitment and prefer to wait for Muslims to take the first step.

Such a deadlock is typical of such situations, in that parties in an active and confrontational conflict are unlikely to take the initiative in seeking reconciliation, or instead may demand too much of the other side before they accept participation in a process initiated by others. To break the cycle and gradually push those on both sides who are most invested in the conflict toward a serious engagement of the process of reconciliation, one should look to other forces and institutions in society. That role could be played by enlightened religious or community leaders, but it is often young people who take the lead in such efforts.

I would therefore call for engaging institutions of higher education in the processes of reducing tensions and encouraging dialogue. These institutions are best suited for this task for several reasons. For example, the diversity of the student body in colleges and universities is conductive to cross-cultural and inter-religious dialogue. As students of different ethnic, religious, and cultural backgrounds get to know each other, they tend to realize and appreciate that they have more in common as human beings than what appears to divide them. The academic environment is also conducive to dialogue because it exposes students to different cultures and ideologies and challenges their assumptions about their own societies and its institutions. Such influences are usually most productive in the minds and souls of young people who have not yet become invested in narrow self-interest or tied down by obligations of family and community.

However, higher education is unlikely to play such a useful role in breaking the deadlock of conflicts like 9/11 and its aftermath without strong and visionary leadership from the faculty and administration of its institutions. That leadership is critical for encouraging and guiding students in the direction of reconciliation. However, unlike their young and fresh students, faculty and administration personnel can themselves be part of the problem because of their own bias or experiences, or at least be distracted by different considerations. But that tendency can be countered by a strong vision of the educational mission that has to be developed over time, rather than expected to suddenly emerge in a time of crisis.

This necessary vision of the educational mission in the service of reconciliation at all levels should include a commitment to integrate international perspectives in the curricular and extracurricular activities so as to better prepare students for life in this age of intense and accelerated globalization. It is particularly important in this regard to encourage and support students and faculty to integrate a commitment to positive social change in academic and scholarly work. A good example of this approach to scholarship in the service of positive social change can be seen in the work of the Law and Religion Program of Emory University throughout the 1990s, and more recently under the auspices of the Center for the Interdisciplinary Study of Religion.[18] With the strong support of those programs, the Ford Foundation, and the university administration, the Religion and Human Rights Project implemented a series of projects over the next six years to address issues of women's access to and control over land in Africa and questions of Islamic Family Law.[19] The current work of this project is a Fellowship Program in Islam and Human Rights, which consists of training and support for human rights advocates in Islamic societies and establishing a permanent web-based resource for scholars and activists in this field.[20] As these activities clearly illustrate, a university can develop and support initiatives for positive social change with scholarly vigor and political independence.

In Sudan, my country of origin, there is a proverb that can be translated as saying: "You should feed your donkey all the time, not only when you need to ride it." In the same way that we need to invest in the normative and institutional resources for justice and accountability to support the process of reconciliation in general, we need to invest in enlightened and responsible education that includes faculty and administrators as well as students.

Notes

1. Al-Kaya al-Harasiy, *Ahkam al-Qur'an* (The Precepts of the Qur'an) (Beirut: al-Muktabah al-'ilmiya, 1983), vol. 1, pp. 78–89.

2. Several parties to that civil war claimed religious justification for their political positions, until one side prevailed and established the Amaway dynasty, which ruled from 661 to 750. The rebellion that succeeded in overthrowing that dynasty and established the Abbasy dynasty also claimed a religious rationale. On that period in Islamic history, see, for example, Wilferd Madelung, *The Succession of Muhammad: A Study of the Early Caliphate* (Cambridge: Cambridge University Press, 1997), chapter 4.

3. Abdullahi Ahmed An-Na'im, "Islamic Ambivalence to Political Violence: Islamic Law and International Terrorism," *German Yearbook of International Law*, vol. 31 (1988), pp. 307–336.

4. Muhammad Hamidullah, *The Muslim Conduct of State* (Lahore, Pakistan: Sh. M. Ashraf, 1966), pp. 305–309.

5. Khaled Abou El Fadl, *Rebellion and Violence in Islamic Law* (Cambridge: Cambridge University Press, 2001), pp. 337–342.

6. See, for example, John W. Whitehead, "Anti-Terrorism Legislation and the Domestic Protection of Human Rights," *American University Law Review*, vol. 51 (August 2002), pp. 1081–1133; and Amnesty International, "United States of America: Amnesty International's concerns regarding post September 11 detentions in the USA," AI-index: 51/044/2002, 14/03/2002, available at www.web.amnesty.org, viewed October 4, 2002.

7. *The Washington Post*, September 5, 2002, p. A31.

8. John Paul Lederach, *Preparing for Peace: Conflict Transformation Across Cultures* (Syracuse, NY: Syracuse University Press, 1995), p. 17.

9. Mahmood Mamdani, "Introduction," in Mahmood Mamdani and Ernest Wamba-dia-Wamba, eds., *African Studies in Social Movements and Democracy* (Dakar, Senegal: CODESRIA, 1995), pp. 9–10.

10. See, for example, www.nytimes.com/ref/nationchallenged/text-index.html for major news stories and analysis on the first anniversary of 9/11.

11. Article 7(1) of the Rome Statute of the International Criminal Court of 1998. U.N. Doc. 32/A/CONF. 183/9, 37 I.L.M. 999.

12. Principles of International Co-Operation in the Detection, Arrest, Extradition and Punishment of Persons Guilty of War Crimes and Crimes Against Humanity, adopted by the UN General Assembly, on December 3, 1973. G.A. Res. 3074, 28th Sess. Supp. No. 30, at 78.

13. Article 14 of the International Covenant on Civil and Political Rights of 1966. 999 U.N.T.S. 171, 6 I.L.M. 368 (1967).

14. Declaration on Principles of International Law Concerning Friendly Relations and Co-Operation Among States in Accordance with the Charter of the United Nations of 1970. G.A. Res. 2625 (XXXV) 25 GAOR, Supp. (No. 28) 121; reprinted in 9 I.L.M. 1292 (1970). These principles are also provided for by Article 2(3) and (4) of the Charter of the United Nations.

15. In addition to sources cited in the preceding paragraph, see, for example, "Fundamental Rules of International Humanitarian Law Applicable in Armed Conflicts," *International Review of the Red Cross* 248 (Geneva: International Committee of the Red Cross, 1978).

16. For further elaboration and documentation of this possibility, see, for example, Laura A. Dickinson, "Using Legal Process to Fight Terrorism: Detentions, Military Commissions, International Tribunals, and the Rule of Law," *Southern California Law Review*, vol. 75, pp. 1407–1492.

17. The Security Council adopted two resolutions prior to the beginning of that campaign on October 7. In Resolution 1368 of September 12, 2001, the Council simply condemned the attacks of 9/11, and "decided to remain seized of the matter," without making any other decision. Resolution 1373 of 28 September 2001 affirmed the right of self-defense in its preamble, but did not sanction any use of force under Chapter VII of the Charter of the United Nations.

18. For an overview of these groundbreaking scholarly and educational initiatives, see, for example, www.law.emory.edu/cisr.

19. These studies are available at www.law.emory.edu/WAL and www.law.emory.edu/IFL. Three books have already been published in 2002 and 2003 by Zed Books, London, out of these studies: Abdullahi A. An-Na'im, ed., *Cultural Transformation and Human Rights in Africa*; L. Muthoni Wanyeki, ed., *Women and Land in Africa: Culture, Religion and Realizing Women's Rights*; Abdullahi A. An-Na'im, ed., *Islamic Family Law in a Changing World: A Global Resource Book.*

20. See www.law.emory.edu/IHR.

Reconciliation in the
New Millennium

Jimmy Carter

When I accepted the Nobel Peace Prize in 2002, I reflected on the fact that instead of entering a millennium of peace, the world is now, in many ways, a more dangerous place than it was in the last century. The greater ease of travel and communication has not been matched by equal understanding and mutual respect. There is a plethora of civil wars, unrestrained by the rules of the Geneva Convention, within which an overwhelming portion of the casualties are unarmed civilians who have no ability to defend themselves. And recent appalling acts of terrorism have reminded us that no nation, even a superpower, is invulnerable. Given this state of affairs, how can we begin to conceive of reconciliation in conflicts so volatile and intractable?

As Wayne Booth notes in the introduction to this volume, reconciliation is a word with abundant meanings, ranging from mending a severed friendship, to ending conflict, to balancing financial accounts. As different as these definitions are, all imply a previous relationship, whether it is one of friendship, of enmity, or even something less personal. The greatest challenge for reconciliation that we face, and the greatest tragedy in our day, is when there is no relationship. How can we hope to achieve reconciliation, to bring together estranged parties, when such a gulf exists that they have no contact with each other at all?

Such a chasm exists between the relatively wealthy and the poor people of this earth. Most of the time, those blessed with prosperity write the existence of the poverty-stricken out of our consciousness, and we proceed with self-satisfaction and a sense of pride in our own good fortune, firmly believing that we have this good fortune because we deserve it. When the Nobel Committee asked me to discuss the greatest challenge facing the world today, I chose this very chasm between the rich and the poor. Citizens of the ten wealthiest countries are now seventy-five times richer than those who live in the ten poorest ones, and the separation is increasing every year—not only between nations but within them. The results of this disparity are the root causes of most of the world's problems, including starvation, illiteracy, environmental degradation, violent conflict, and unnecessary illness. There are 1.2 billion people on earth living on less than one dollar per day for food, shelter, clothing, medicine (if it is available), and education (if it is available). They live without any sanitation, without fresh, clean water, without any prospect of the next meal. And we do not even know they exist.

One of our projects at the Carter Center analyzes all the conflicts on earth. There are more now than ever before in history: our list shows about 110 in an average year. About seventy of these erupt into violence each year. And of these seventy or so violent conflicts, about thirty become what we call a major war, which is a war in which at least 1,000 soldiers have been killed on the battlefield; almost all of these are civil wars. In these wars, for every soldier who perishes, nine civilians die from stray bombs, bullets, missiles, or from the deliberate deprivation of food and shelter. And we in the United States are rarely involved in a constructive way in preventing those conflicts, either as individuals or through government or universities.

Since I left office over twenty years ago, the United States has launched military attacks against twelve nations, sometimes with horrendous loss of life, and with almost total impunity for our own military forces—for which I am thankful, having served in the Navy for twelve years. Such conflicts can be tempting to a leader in the White House or the Department of Defense—they produce great admiration of these leaders, who become the commanders of our young men and women in danger overseas rather than just civilian administrators. But my opinion is that very few, if any, of the military attacks in the past twenty years were justified. In most cases, they were caused by a lack of understanding between people, and also, quite often, a lack of understanding by our own leaders of the peculiar circumstances that caused the conflict or the motivations or promises or psychological attitudes or background or history or political commitments of the leaders involved. An analysis of the cause of conflicts—both past and potentially in the future—and how certain elements of mediation might have prevented them would be a very fruitful effort.

Within our own country, as other essays in this volume address, recurring conflicts stem from a history of what amounted to apartheid in the United States. From the time I was four years old until I left home to go to the Naval Academy, I lived on a farm in south Georgia, which I have written about recently in *An Hour Before Daylight: Memories of a Rural Boyhood*. Much of my childhood took place during the Great Depression, when my family lived in abject poverty. There were millions of people from the North who moved to the South, having lost their jobs because factories closed or were modernized. We would have two or three hundred so-called hoboes go by in front of our house every day, some quite well educated, looking for anything—a drink of cold water, or maybe a sandwich or piece of chicken leg left over from dinner. The highest level of living for most families was to be a sharecropper, with the right to support one's family on roughly thirty-five acres of land. The average yearly income of a sharecropper family then was seventy-five dollars. Black and white people were brought close together because of this shared poverty.

Our country lived for about a hundred years—from the time of the Civil War until the Civil Rights Movement—under Supreme Court rulings that said separate but equal was the law of the land. But we were neither separate nor equal. I did not know what separate meant, because I lived on a farm with no white neighbors; I played with and fought with and wrestled with and fished with and worked with only black children, African American kids. And we were certainly not equal, though we considered ourselves to be basically so. I am ashamed to admit that in those days, I never realized the deprivation of their lives compared to mine. It did not bother me, I hate to admit, that their parents could not vote, could not serve on a jury, that they could not go to a decent school, and that, if we rode to Americus together (the county seat), my playmates sat in the colored section and I sat in the white section. That system prevailed in our country for a hundred years. There was no white liberal or black activist who demanded that the Supreme Court change its basic ruling. The visitors who came to our little church in Plains even supported that premise with selected verses from the Holy Scriptures.

Under today's laws, we are legally equal but we have become separate again. For the Atlanta Project at the Carter Center, I visited every high school in the Atlanta area, and I was pained to see that at one school in southwest Atlanta with 850 students, not a single one was white. In the debate over whether we should do away with affirmative action, one side argues that it is a liberal give-away program that deprives white kids of their chance at college. What those on this side of the argument forget is that the inherent ravages of slavery remain, and result in the deliberate legal deprivation of African American children's basic right to a decent education.

Reconciliation is difficult to originate among those who are deprived. It has to come from above, from the elite who make the decisions and shape the ideas and inspire people who are in positions of power. And there is no source of that inspiration or that study or that free analysis that can equal a university campus, where there is a diversity of views and absolute guaranteed freedom of expression, and hopefully an innovative attitude toward the problems that present themselves.

On the afternoon in 2000 before I spoke to a symposium on reconciliation at Emory University, I participated in a press conference that presented a new concept for the Georgia flag. I was very proud of what the Georgia House of Representatives did that day. But being there also reminded me of how much things have changed since I was governor in the early 1970s. One thing that came to mind was the way we treat one of the most deprived constituencies in our country—that is, those convicted of a crime. In those days, there was an intense competition between me and the governors of Florida, Alabama, Arkansas, Tennessee, South Carolina, and North Carolina about who could reduce the prison population most. I organized volunteer probation officers—members of the Lions Clubs, Kiwanis Clubs, Rotary Clubs, and so forth—who would say, "I will take one parolee and be responsible for him." The parolee would most often be a young black man, and the volunteer probation officer would most often be a white man. The officer had to pledge his word of honor that he would visit the parolee's family before he was released, that he would find a job for that young man, take responsibility for him as though he were his own.

Today, there seems to be a competition among governors over who can build the most prison cells and who can keep people incarcerated the longest. When California adopted the "three strikes, you're out" rule—meaning that if you have three felony convictions, most often possession of drugs, you serve the rest of your life in prison—Georgia played one-upmanship and adopted a "two strikes, you're out" rule. When I was governor, and when I was president, there were no people in this country executed. Now there are more than 3,000 people on Death Row; on some days there are two or three people executed on the same day. There never has been and never will be a rich white man or woman executed in this country. Because of policies that we all condone or accept, the people who are executed are those too poverty-stricken to have a competent lawyer, or who are a minority, or who are mentally retarded.

Some say that these chasms among the haves and have-nots cannot be bridged in a nation as inherently divided as ours. While people point to the 2000 presidential election campaign as evidence that this country is as divided as it has ever been, I believe that is a misconception. What that election showed us is that our country is divided almost equally, but in superficial ways, comparatively speaking. If you consider the Civil War, the Civil Rights Movement, or the Vietnam War, you see a country truly divided. Today, you need the subtle analysis of a political scientist to see the difference between the Republican position and the Democratic position. There are some differences, but they are not profound. We have a united nation, in other words. While the post–September 11 world presents enormous challenges, we also have a chance to set national goals that are exalting, or inspirational, or profoundly significant. I have been in politics for a long time—in the State Senate, governorship, and the White House—and I can tell you that the chance that that sort of inspiration and new ideas will come from within the political community is unlikely. This is not a criticism of politicians, but rather a realistic view of how politics works. So, where is the potential origin of new concepts of justice and fairness? I would argue that it is in the great universities of our country.

When I left office, I gave a farewell address; one of the lines that I used was that I was graduating from the White House to the highest position that can be held by a human being in America: private citizen. The policies of our government are shaped by the private citizens of this country, those who have the freedom to think and to consider and to assess what is done in our own nation, and around the world, and to try to extract from those considerations a finer way, a better way, to resolve some of our problems.

The theologian Reinhold Niebuhr says that the highest possible calling of an organization like a government is to establish justice in a sinful world. The highest calling of a human being, he says, is to practice love—unselfish love, or *agape*, to use the Greek word. This means that there is an inherent limit on exaltation or aspirations or goals or priorities between the government and any individual citizen. Collectively, though, we citizens can change the concept of our nation. It does not take many. All it takes is a few professors or students in a law school or a theology school, or a few professors or students studying sociology or political science—a few people who are aware of what goes on in the world and the need to improve people's circumstances, and who can then propose a better way to do things. And we do need to turn to doing things, to taking action.

One of the most difficult things for any human being is to address a complicated question and to have new ideas truly above and beyond what has already been done. The universities in our country are places where such thinking can happen. One sterling characteristic of American life that is not challenged anywhere on earth is the quality of our system of higher education. Our universities are a special treasure. I believe that this treasure can be a source of inspiration for those working on justice in our neighborhoods and around the globe. Our universities are a key component in achieving reconciliation.

If we encourage it, the university can be a place where students learn many different, and even unorthodox, ways of solving problems. Furthermore, while it is helpful to theorize about an important issue like reconciliation, we also need to pay attention to actions. At the Carter Center, we have programs that involve sixty-five nations in the world; thirty-five of those countries—generally the poorest countries on earth—are in Africa. And although the greatness of American universities is universally recognized, we rarely if ever see any indication in those countries of the existence of an American university. And even when an American university is present, that presence is not felt by the people. Too often, this enormous treasure that we have in our country is absorbed with its own self-interest, pursuing academic programs, studying in a desiccated way the activities and perhaps even on occasion the plight of others whom we do not know. Crossing those chasms of ignorance or willful blindness is particularly important now, in light of the challenges of globalism and the threat of continued international conflict.

Will the brains and resources and innovative spirit and freedom found in our higher educational institutions be exerted to find some solutions to the problems that I have described briefly? I think we can move toward reconciliation if we try to answer a question that is both very simple and very complex: How do we—in the name of justice and peace, freedom, democracy, human rights, and the alleviation of suffering—break down the barriers between ourselves and others?

An Agenda for Higher Education

Rebecca S. Chopp

To celebrate the turning of a new millennium, I initiated a cross-disciplinary symposium at Emory University on diverse approaches to reconciliation. As the then-provost of that institution, which is home to a leading school of theology and linked to the Carter Center, discussion of this topic seemed an appropriate way to begin the twenty-first century. The terrorist attacks of September 11, 2001, and their aftermath brought the conversation about political and cultural reconciliation, in particular, into sharp relief.

The diversity and complexity of conflicts in this new era, like the diversity of approaches to conflicts in this volume, render any single "grand narrative" of reconciliation impossible.[1] We cannot have one shared, common understanding of how all the pieces of such a complex process in so many cultural locations can fit together. To strive for an all-encompassing narrative would be to repress voices, to stop evolutionary processes, to fix things that could not and should not be fixed. The diversity of approaches to understanding reconciliation in the essays in this volume instead sketches a picture of what it means to take reconciliation seriously in the context of higher education. In this country newly wakened from the dream of invulnerability to terror, from the false sleep of isolation from the chronic global problems, the role of higher education in preparing citizens is more vital than ever. As Thomas Jefferson said, "I know of no safe repository of the ultimate powers of the society but the people themselves; and if we think them not enlightened enough to exercise control with a wholesome discretion, the remedy is not to take it from them, but to inform their discretion by education."[2]

Education and citizenship have traveled together throughout the history of the United States. As historian Thomas Bender has shown,

America's earliest institutions of higher learning were civic and public.[3] Across this country, colleges—such as Harvard and Colgate and Duke, and much later Stanford—were founded so that men could be trained for public and church life. So important was training leaders for civic society, a point of great pride was to have a college or an academy. The Morrill Act, a land grant of 1862, extended the notion of education for democracy to rural and agrarian culture. The progressive movement extended education to immigrants in our cities. And the special link between historically black colleges and African American communities ensured that training would be available for those denied citizens, who would soon be in the republic as fully engaged citizens. A simple statistic illustrates this: between 1870 and 1940, the U.S. population tripled, but the number of students in colleges increased thirty times. America has depended upon higher education to strengthen civic society time and time again.

In recent years, though, the fundamental role of education has been shoved aside by the notion of education as preparation for a profession, on one hand, and education as the institution of pure research on the other. Both should be envisioned in new ways in order to further the aims of this democracy. Kept out of perspective, these goals distort the promises and functions of education. Historians of education note that America's unique contribution to education is not that of the research university but that of the liberal arts college. Most fully in America have we realized the goal of education for citizenship and life in general. Liberal arts—alone among the forms of higher education in this country—has clung tenaciously to civic education as a fundamental purpose. From this strong and deep foundation of democracy, we should again retrieve the formation of citizens as a basic goal of higher education.

First, I recommend that leaders in higher education reclaim and revise the purpose of higher education: to create world citizens, no matter what their specific undergraduate or professional school training. The notion that education is fundamentally about creating, forming, or shaping citizens is not a new idea; it is as old as education itself. But it is one that higher education as a whole needs to reclaim and revise if it is to remain vital. In her book *Cultivating Humanity*, Martha Nussbaum links education with the changing nature of what it means to be a world citizen in the twenty-first century: "Many of our most pressing problems require for their intelligent, cooperative solution a dialogue that brings together people from many different national and cultural and religious backgrounds."[4]

Too often, our endeavor is in ragged pieces—disciplines here, projects there, professional schools on the edges. Life on a campus need not be constructed in tight-fitting pieces, but we do need to shape a culture that shows we understand that we share a common vision. We need to prepare people *not* to agree with one another all the time, but to live in a world with the skill and heart and imagination and tools necessary, time and time again, to take on new projects of reconciliation.

At this moment, the relationship between higher education and citizenship is not a part of our conversation about education. And when forming and shaping citizens is not an explicit part of what we do, I fear we slip into an anonymous vision of what we are forming and shaping people for. This problem echoes throughout each essay in this volume's section on higher education. When educators do not understand what we do as connected to the broader world, we risk simply teaching people to go out and live lives that are unreflective, unquestioning, unassuming, unconnected to the natural, social, and global environment around them. Higher education must ensure that this does not happen. Higher education is not only preparation for a job, and the life well lived is not only about the attainment of material goods.

As the essays in this volume make clear, the world now—in crisis environmentally, politically, economically, and socially—requires us to reclaim the role, or even responsibility, of higher education in addressing world problems. But even as we reclaim this heritage, we must revise it. The way of shaping and forming citizens one hundred years ago, fifty years ago, even twenty years ago, is not the way forward. For the formation of citizens today and in the future, we must ask and answer different questions than in the past.

We need to prepare world citizens who can address issues of racism —all forms of racism, as Johnnetta Cole reminds us. We need to revise our education to make sure that our students, with commitment and sophistication, can address the economic injustices in our country; that they understand, with Reverend Joseph Lowery, that all God's children got shoes; that they understand that the world, as Dan Carter and former president Jimmy Carter both remind us, is a world in horribly poor economic condition. We must shape world citizens who can ask and answer very difficult questions about economics and mission, such as the role of entrepreneurship in the university, and who or what controls the research agenda. These are questions for scholars, but they are also questions for students. In a world filled with many different religions, we must understand that now well-worn debates or lack thereof, such as those around religion and science or religion and politics, need to be thought of in new ways. We must form and shape new citizens of the world who will not engage in runaway consumerism and the rampant destruction of our environment.

Learning that prepares students to engage in reconciliation as global citizens means encountering a world that is constantly falling out of place, and setting that world anew, setting the world "aright," as Hannah Arendt wrote. Perhaps now, as never before, her words ring true:

> Basically we are always educating for a world that is out of joint, for this is the basic human situation, in which the world is created by mortal hands to serve mortals for a limited time as home. Because the world is made by mortals it wears out; and because it continuously changes its inhabitants it runs the risk of becoming as mortal as they. To preserve the world against the mortality of its creators and inhabitants it must be constantly set anew. The problem is to educate in such a way that a setting aright remains possible.[5]

Those of us in higher education need to reclaim and revise our educational purpose as one that shapes world citizens who aspire and value, who can and will do the hard work, and who dream of setting the world anew, setting the world aright. And we can do this by cultivating three habits of thought and work and life: critique, truth-telling, and imagination.

Critique

Perhaps the most heartening thread that runs through all the essays in this volume is that, though we value reconciliation, we do not do so blindly. No one wants an easy, cheap form of reconciliation; no one wants reconciliation as smoothing over conflict so that things will be easy again. We want to go forward in the task of reconciliation with a healthy sense of critique. Reconciliation implies that things can be fixed, but it also implies that hard questions can and must be asked—when a theory does not match the facts, when the language of freedom is distorted by the silence of groups of persons, when the disciplines either rub each other so frequently that each is transformed or are so disconnected that bridges in our academic city must be built. To equip students to offer useful critiques as global citizens, we need to help them develop fluency in bridge building, connecting, global travel and communications. Today, this means attending to methods and ways of connecting knowledge, learning different cultures, and relating and managing information.

Students also need a greater degree of literacy in science, humanities, the arts, and social sciences. Citizens of tomorrow, engaged on the world stage of technological, economic, and environmental change, need to be able to acquire information about images of humans, about facts of human culture, and about the natural world. For this, they have to possess a basic literacy of the concepts and practices of thinking and expression in what we know as the liberal arts. True literacy in these arts and fluency in the scientific method consists of an openness of inquiry, the communal character of deliberation, the wiliness to submit hypotheses for public deliberation, and the imagination required for successful practice.[6]

Truth-telling

In recommending that we teach the value of truth-telling, I must again invoke Lyotard: no grand narrative of truth can be offered. But perhaps truth as a utopian quest is how we in the academy become a figure of hope again for our society and for the world. Perhaps truth-telling is always a process—not one of luxury, to borrow the words of Audre Lorde, but one necessary for our survival. Maynard Hutchison may have called this ongoing quest for truth the "great conversation"— the noisy, blooming, buzzing confusion of all the disciplines together, questing after this truth, sorting and re-sorting them out. Reconciliation, as an aspiration for forming and shaping world citizens, must be forged through critique, crafted through the imagination, and anchored always and only in truth.

I am struck by the variety of approaches to truth-telling in reconciliation in this volume: from Tammy Krause's chronicle of the confrontation of victims by the offenders who harmed them to Angelika Bammer's probing of the divisions among Americans who claim to "stand united." From E.O. Wilson's call for a future-oriented, global environmental policy to Abdullahi An-Na'im's call for legal redress of terrorist crimes, the authors make this point: we need a new narrative, for justice, for living with the self, for living together as a society and a world. And this narrative requires a certain amount of truth-telling.

Quite simply, then, as we think about our teaching and our learning, these three habits are serious ones that we have to form and perform in the arts, the sciences, the humanities, and the social sciences. We must strengthen the habit of critique, to ask hard questions; the habit of truth-telling, to have the courage, the conviction, the inner sensibility, to follow where those questions lead; and the habit of imagination, the vision to craft the tools to think in new ways as we remember that reconciliation is never easy and never simple. This is a kind of utopian realist's quest, but it is, I think, how we continue our task of setting the world anew, setting the world aright.

Imagination

The essays on psychological reconciliation by Professors Paul and Fivush illustrate that imagination is necessary for a person to be able to form a narrative that helps him or her move through and past trauma. To educate students for democracy and global citizenship, we too must help them imagine how to move forward from the traumas of history. Developing a sense of historical knowledge and moral imagination is vital to that process. Here, history, religion, philosophy, and art teach how past cultures addressed the problems of their day. Anthropology, psychology, and political science must teach us about the current conditions and ways to model change. We use the traditions, as Hans Georg Gadamer has noted, for new interpretations, new visions, and new practices.[7] We have waffled in recent years in relation to this task, careful to not offend, unsure of how to talk about morality without offending, ill at ease with public debates. But we must use our bonds of community to "remember forward," to imagine new paths of working together, new images of being human together, new conversations of and in our democracy. To quote Emily Dickinson, the "slow fuse" of the "possible" is lit by the imagination. Our task in higher education should be to light the fuse of the possible.

Notes

1. Jean-Francois Lyotard, *The Postmodern Condition: A Report on Knowledge*, 6th ed., trans. Geoff Bennington and Brain Massumi (Minneapolis: University of Minnesota Press, 1988).

2. Thomas Jefferson, letter to William C. Jarvis, September 28, 1820. Jefferson Library. See www.monticello.org.

3. Thomas Bender, *Intellect and Public Life: Essays on the Social History of American Intellectuals in the United States* (Baltimore: Johns Hopkins Press, 1993).

4. Martha C. Nussbaum, *Cultivating Humanity: A Classical Defense of Reform in Liberal Education* (Cambridge, MA: Harvard University Press, 1997).

5. Hannah Arendt, "The Crisis of Education," in *Between Past and Future: Eight Exercises in Political Thought* (New York: Viking Press, 1961).

6. Richard J. Bernstein, "John Dewey on Democracy: The Task Before Us," *Philosophical Profiles: Essays in a Pragmatic Mode* (Philadelphia: University of Pennsylvania Press, 1986), p. 272.

7. Hans Georg Gadamer, *Truth and Method* (New York: Seabury Press, 1975).

About the Contributors

Abdullahi Ahmed An-Na'im is Charles Howard Candler Professor of Law at Emory University and director of the Religion and Human Rights Program. He is an internationally recognized scholar of Islam and human rights in cross-cultural perspectives whose research interests also include constitutionalism in Islamic and African countries, and Islam and politics.

Angelika Bammer is a professor in the Institute for Liberal Arts at Emory University. She is the author of *Partial Visions: Feminism and Utopianism in the 1970s* (1991), and is currently at work on a book titled *Memory Work: Constructing Histories, Producing Pasts.*

Wayne Booth is George M. Pullman Distinguished Service Professor, Emeritus, at the University of Chicago. His publications include *The Rhetoric of Fiction* (1961, 1983), *Modern Dogma and the Rhetoric of Dissent* (1974), and *The Company We Keep: An Ethics of Fiction* (1988).

Amy Benson Brown is director of the Manuscript Development Program at Emory University and author of *Rewriting the Word: American Women Writers and the Bible* (1998). She is currently working on a book about the nineteenth-century activist Sarah Moore Grimké.

Dan Carter is Educational Foundation University Professor at the University of South Carolina. His publications include *The Politics of Rage: George Wallace, the Origins of the New Conservatism, and the Transformation of American Politics* (2000) and *Scottsboro: A Tragedy of the American South* (1990).

Jimmy Carter was the thirty-ninth president of the United States. After leaving office, he established the Carter Center in Atlanta, Georgia, and authored numerous books on history and the challenges of peacemaking, faith, and aging. The Carter Center seeks to prevent and resolve international conflicts, enhance freedom and democracy, and improve world health. In 2002, he was awarded the Nobel Peace Prize for his decades of work to promote peace, democracy, human rights, and economic development throughout the world.

Rebecca S. Chopp is president of Colgate University and president of the American Academy of Religion. A former provost at Emory University, her publications include *The Power to Speak: Feminism, Language, and God* (1989) and *Saving Work: Feminist Practices of Theological Education* (1995).

Johnnetta B. Cole served as president of Spelman College from 1987 to 1997 and currently serves as president of Bennett College. She has edited *Anthropology for the Nineties* (1988) and is the author of *Conversations: Straight Talk with America's Sister President* (1994).

Robyn Fivush is a professor of psychology at Emory University whose research focuses on memory, children, and trauma. Her publications include *The Remembering Self: Construction and Accuracy in the Life Narrative* (ed. with U. Neisser, 1994) and *Children's Recollections of Traumatic and Non-traumatic Experiences* (1998).

Tammy Krause works with victims outreach for the Arizona Federal Public Defender. She is former director of JustBridges, a program that builds working relationships between victims and defense attorneys, and she has taught in the Justice, Peace, and Conflict Studies Program at Eastern Mennonite University.

Gary Laderman is associate professor of religion at Emory University and author of *Rest in Peace: A Cultural History of Death and the Funeral Home in Twentieth-Century America* (Oxford University Press, 2003) and co-editor of *Religion and American Cultures: An Encyclopedia of Traditions, Diversity, and Popular Expressions* (ABC—Clio, 2003).

Congressman John Lewis, who represents Georgia's fifth district, has written *Walking with the Wind: A Memoir of the Movement* (Harcourt, 1999).

Reverend Joseph E. Lowery is one of the co-founders of the Southern Christian Leadership Conference and was instrumental in the Civil Rights Movement as well as the anti-apartheid movement in the United States.

Richard C. Martin is professor of religion at Emory University. Among his books are *Approaches to Islam in Religious Studies* (1985), *Islamic Studies: A History of Religions Approach* (1996), and *Defenders of Reason in Islam: Mu'tazilism from Medieval School to Modern Symbol* (1997).

Barbara Patterson is senior lecturer in religion at Emory University. An advocate of "scholar citizenship" for faculty and students, she facilitates workshops, programs, and community partnerships in experiential and community-based learning. Committed to the scholarship of teaching, she has published numerous articles on these topics.

Robert A. Paul is Candler Professor in the Graduate Institute of Liberal Arts at Emory University and Dean of Emory College. His publications include *The Tibetan Symbolic World* (1982) and *Moses and Civilization* (1996).

Karen M. Poremski is assistant professor of English at Ohio Wesleyan University. She served as the coordinator of Emory University's Reconciliation Symposium.

Theophus Smith, an ordained minister in the Episcopal Church, is associate professor of religion at Emory University and co-author of *Curing Violence: Essays on Rene Girard* (1994).

Frans B.M. de Waal is Charles Howard Candler Professor of Primate Behavior at Emory University. His publications include *Peacemaking Among Primates* (1989), *Bonobo: The Forgotten Ape* (1997), and *Chimpanzee Politics* (2000).

E.O. Wilson is University Research Professor and Honorary Curator in Entomology at Harvard University. His publications include *On Human Nature* (1978) and *The Ants* (with Bert Hölldobler, 1990), both of which won the Pulitzer Prize for nonfiction, and *Consilience: The Unity of Knowledge* (1998).

Index